Overnight Colon and Liver Cleanse & Detox

Get Your Energy, Stamina and Mental Clarity Back in 11 days and Lose Weight Fast in the Process!

DISCLAIMER

SUMMARY

A detox diet can prove to be very healthy as it provides nutrients to the body which helps remove toxins from the system. A detox diet if carried out appropriately will improve your sense of well-being and increase energy levels by cleansing your body from the inside.

If you are looking for detox diet recipes for the colon and liver, look no farther!

This eBook presents to you exactly what you are looking for!

Prepare yourself to find 50 overnight liver and colon, cleanse and detox diet recipes in this book. These are easy to prepare recipes which will prove beneficial for your overall health. This eBook includes recipes for juices as well as lunch meals to benefit from during your liver and colon detox diet. At a glance, here is what this eBook will benefit you with:

1. 50 overnight detox and cleanse diet recipes for liver and colon
2. Recipes for juices and lunchtime which are easy to prepare
3. A step by step preparation guide to help you easily prepare the recipe
4. A complete nutritional fact sheet of every recipe
5. Serving size and cooking time for every recipe to help you manage the time and ingredients well.

Table of Contents

Introduction

An overnight liver and colon detox diet helps you to flush the toxins from your system, which may have accumulated over the years. Successfully detoxifying the liver and colon helps to restore these vital organs. When your liver is clean of toxins, it will help bowel movements occur more regularly and purify blood.

To follow this overnight liver and colon detox diet you will have to follow the following steps. Remember, that the cleansing occurs overnight but it requires preparation and steps afterwards to ensure maximum success of your detox diet.

Phase One

Phase one includes preparing yourself for the detoxification, and this phase lasts for seven days. Your day should start by consuming a detox drink. You can choose to make any detox drink from recipes given below for each of seven days. You have to have 3 cups of detox juice for breakfast, but you can divide it to drink in intervals.

For example, gulp down one cup as you wake up. Have the second cup of juice after two hours, and before you sit down for lunch, have your third cup of detox juice an hour before lunch.

For lunch and dinner, you must limit your meals to proteins and salads. You may have 3 to 4 servings of food in a day, which is ideal. Lunch and dinner recipes are provided in this eBook and you can swap the recipes between different days of the diet. There is no restriction to having a particular recipe on a particular day. All recipes are detox friendly.

Phase Two

Phase two contains the main event of the detox diet and it is one day long. The most significant detoxification will occur now, once you have prepared your body for it. In this phase, you are required to drink one glass of detox drink every hour alternating it with water. (The recipes are provided below).

For example, if you drink a cup of detox juice at 8 A.M, you will drink a glass of water at 9 A.M. after the next hour, at 10 A.M you will again have a cup of detox juice and keep alternating in this way between water and juice for the entire day. At the end of the day, you will be officially done with your detox diet.

Phase Three

This is the transitional phase, which will last for three days. You will follow the same rules given in phase one, with one exception. Add yogurt to your diet, at least once a day (in lunch or dinner).

After the three days have passed, you can go back to eating normal again, but make sure it is healthy!

Detox Drink Recipes

GREEN PROTEIN SMOOTHIE

SERVING SIZE

1 to 2 persons

COOKING TIME

5 MINUTES

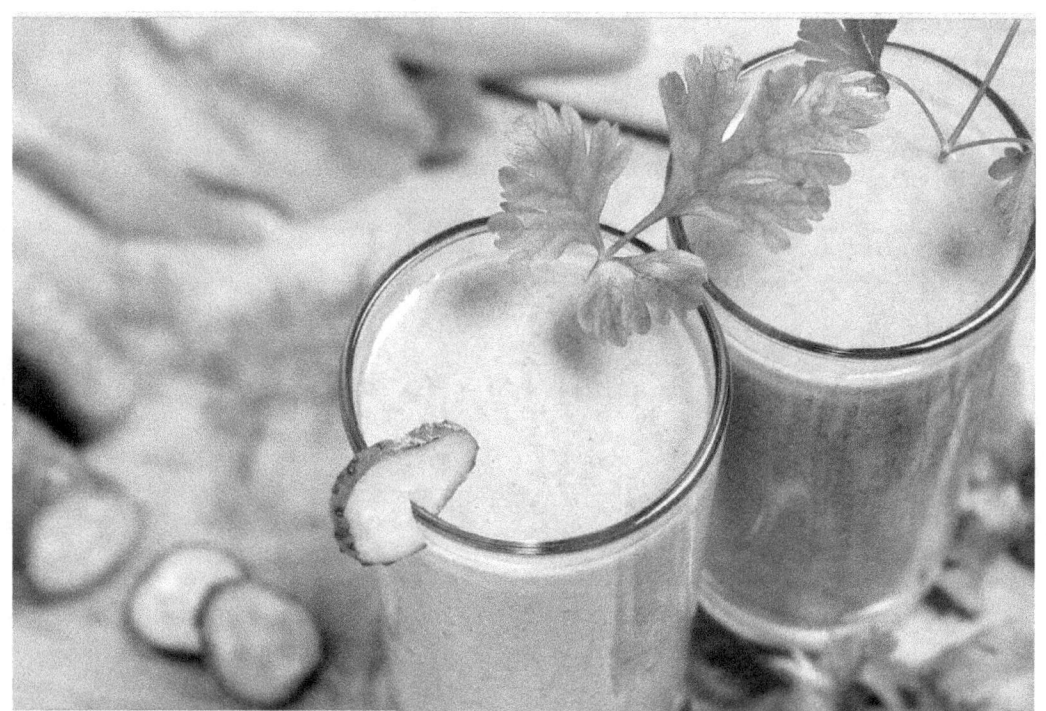

INGREDIENTS

¼ cup diced avocado

½ cup kale

½ tablespoon honey

½ cup spinach

½ cup frozen blueberries

1/3 cup non-fat yoghurt

PREPARATION METHOD

1. Blend ingredients until smooth
2. Serve chilled

NUTRITIONAL VALUE PER SERVING

Calories: 220

Fat: 8g

Protein: 11g

Carbohydrates: 32g

STRAWBERRY SMOOTHIE

SERVING SIZE

1 person

COOKING TIME

5 minutes

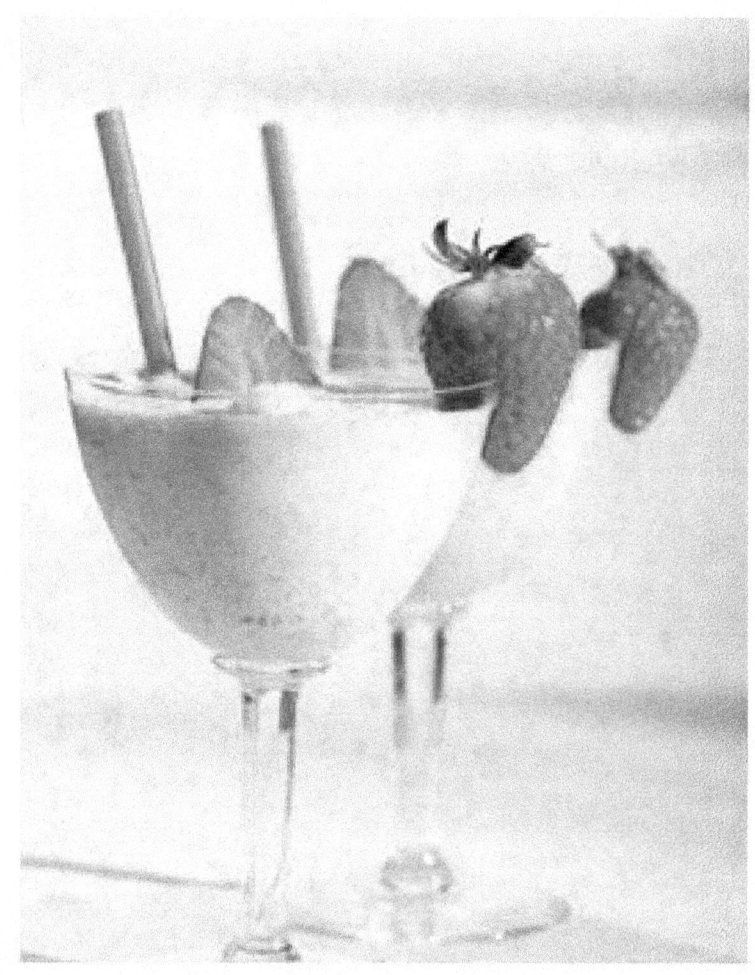

INGREDIENTS

1 banana

3 cups water

8 strawberries

1 tbsp agave nectar

PREPARATION METHOD

1. Add all ingredients in a blender
2. Stir and serve chilled.

NUTRIENT VALUE PER SERVING

Calories: 300

Fat: 1.5g

Carbohydrates: 65g

Protein: 6g

MANGO SMOOTHIE

SERVING SIZE

1 person

COOKING TIME

10 minutes

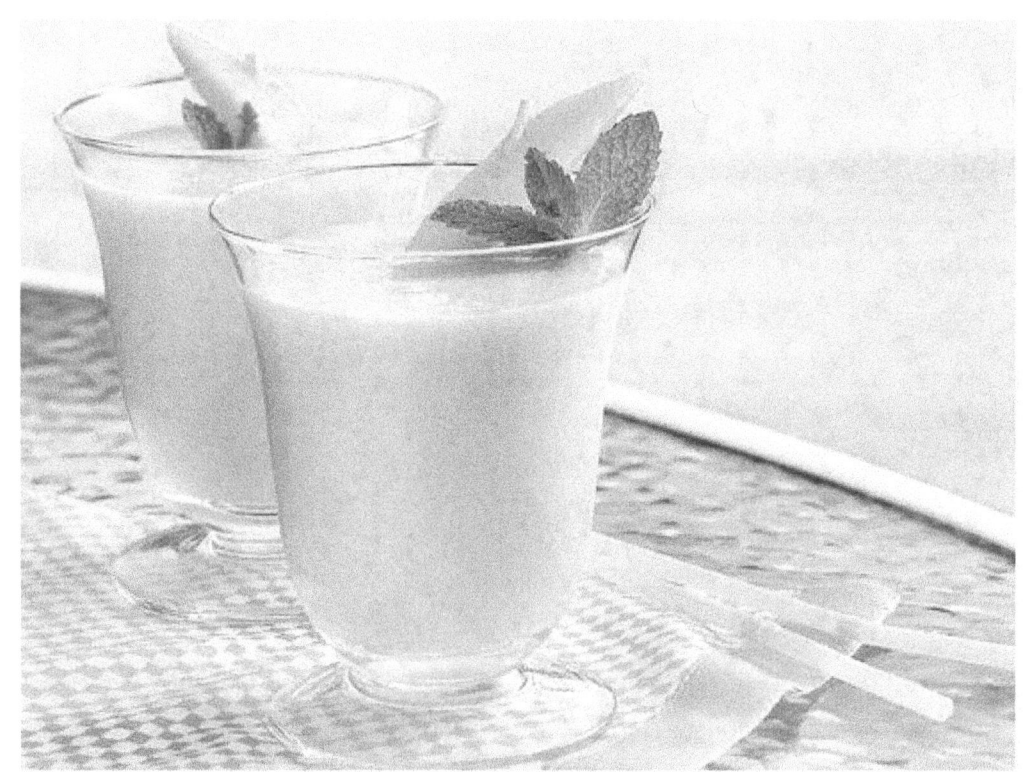

INGREDIENTS

1 ¼ cup almond milk

½ cup coconut water

2 leaves kale (chopped)

¼ avocado

½ cup mango chunks

½ cup ice

PREPARATION METHOD

1. Blend ingredients until smooth
2. Serve chilled

NUTRIENT VALUE PER SERVING

Calories: 360

Fat: 0g

Carbohydrates: 0g

Protein: 0g

CUCUMBER KIWI GREEN SMOOTHIE

SERVING SIZE

One person

COOKING TIME

3-5 minutes

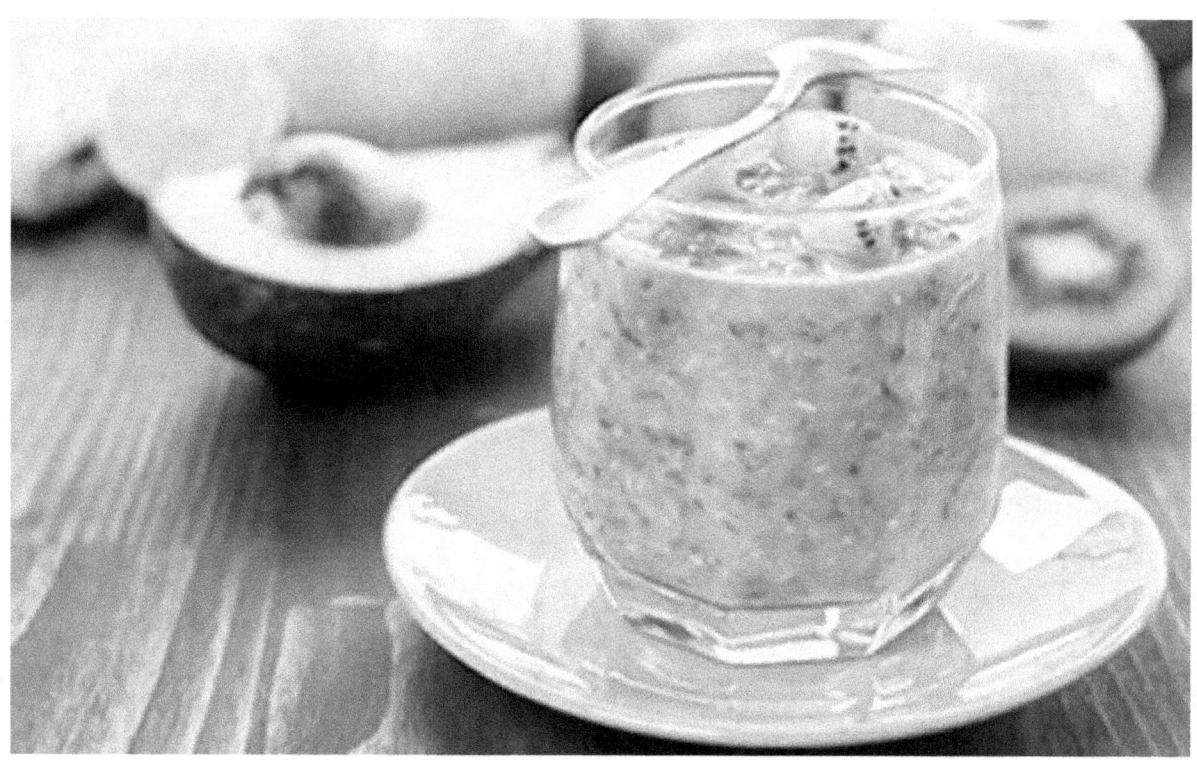

INGREDIENTS

1 peeled cucumber

3 peeled kiwifruits

1 cored apple

3 leaves of Swiss chard

8 ounce unsweetened milk

PREPARATION METHOD

1. Blend the ingredients in water and put in the greens last
2. Serve chilled

NUTRIENT VALUE PER SERVING

Calories: 328

Fat: 2g

Carbohydrates: 72 g

Protein: 9g

PAPAYA PINEAPPLE SMOOTHIE

SERVING SIZE

1 person

COOKING TIME

5 minutes

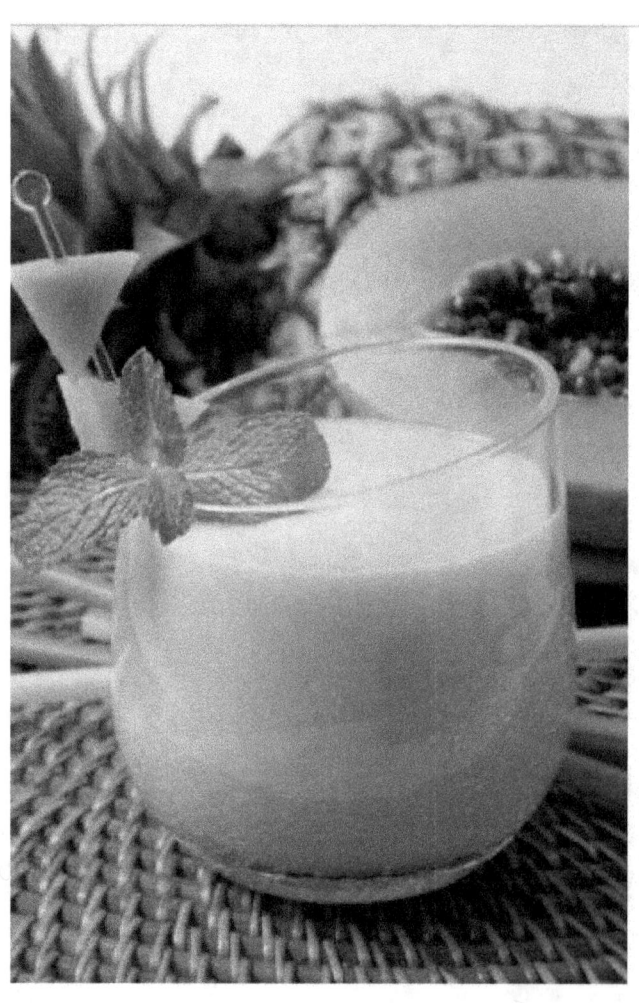

INGREDIENTS

½ cup papaya

½ cup pineapple

¼ cup pineapple juice

¼ cup milk

PREPARATION METHOD

1. Blend all ingredients together and serve chilled.

NUTRIENT VALUE PER SERVING

Calories: 120

Fat: 0.2g

Carbohydrates: 28.3g

Protein: 3.1g

LEMONADE CLEANSE

SERVING SIZE

1 person

COOKING TIME

5 minutes

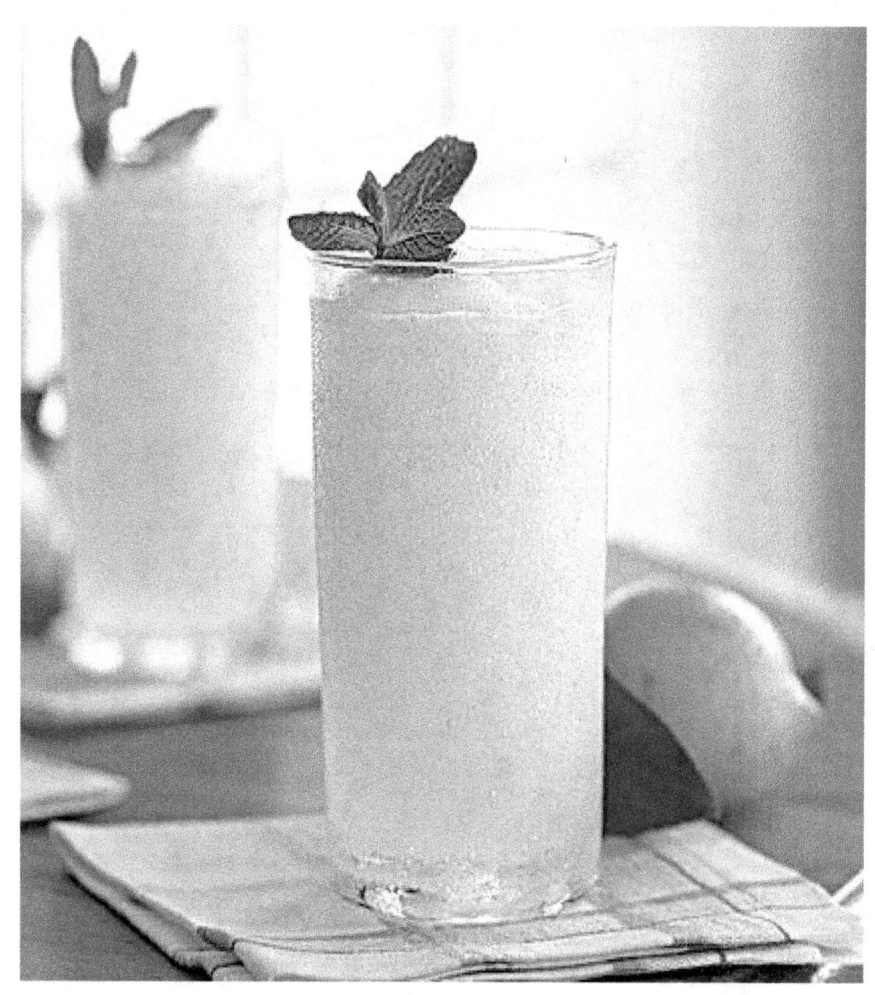

INGREDIENTS

2 tablespoons of lemon juice

2 tablespoons of pure maple syrup

One-tenth teaspoon of cayenne pepper

8 ounces of purified water

PREPARATION METHOD

1. Mix all the ingredients together
2. Serve it chilled

NUTRITIONAL VALUE (PER SERVING)

Calories: 99

Carbohydrates: 25.8g

Protein: 0.2g

Fat: 0.1g

FRESH CRANBERRY JUICE

SERVING SIZE

1 person

PREPARATION TIME

5 minutes

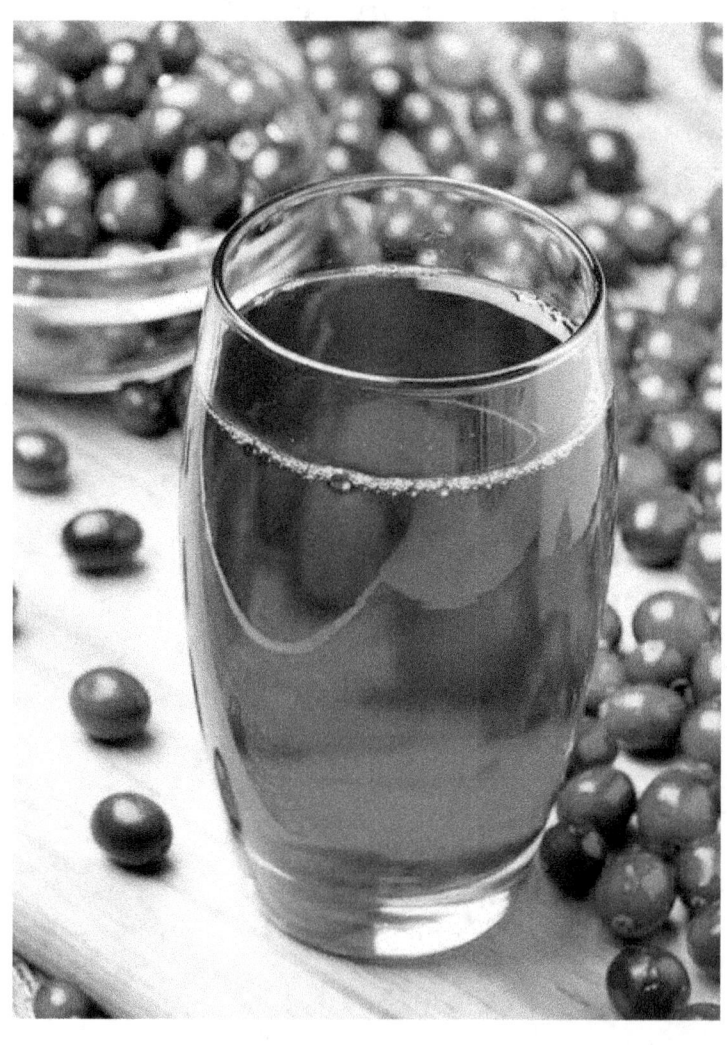

INGREDIENTS

Fresh cranberry juice

Water

1 tablespoon apple pectin

1 tablespoon psyllium fiber

PREPARATION METHOD

1. Dilute one part of cranberry juice with 4 parts of water
2. Add apple pectin and psyllium fiber
3. It is ready to serve

NUTRITIONAL VALUE PER SERVING

Calories: 116

Fat: 0g

Carbohydrates: 31g

Protein: 1g

FRUIT DETOX DRINK:

SERVING SIZE

2 persons

COOKING TIME

5-10 minutes

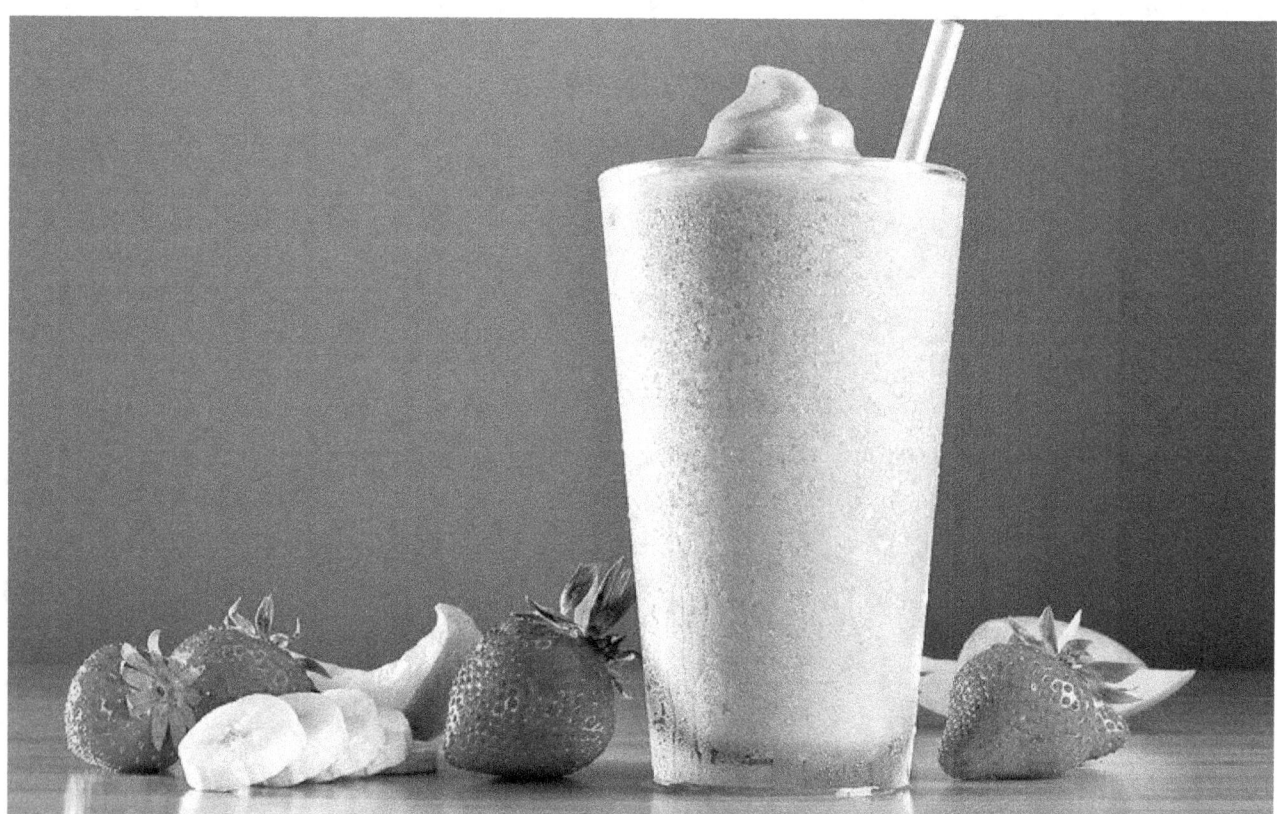

INGREDIENTS

½ cup banana, strawberries or yogurt

½-inch slice of ginger

1 small garlic clove

1 tablespoon flax oil

1 tablespoon freshly squeezed lemon juice if desired

1 tablespoon lecithin granules

1 tablespoon of protein powder or spirulina powder

4 oz. of pure water

8 oz. of orange juice

PREPARATION METHOD

1. Add all the ingredients in blender and mix until smooth.
2. Serve as chilled as you like.

NUTRITIONAL VALUE PER SERVING

Calories: 108

Fat: 0.35g

Carbohydrates: 29.18g

Protein: 0.98g

BEETROOT, CARROT AND APPLE DETOX JUICE

SERVING SIZE

1 person

COOKING TIME

10 minutes

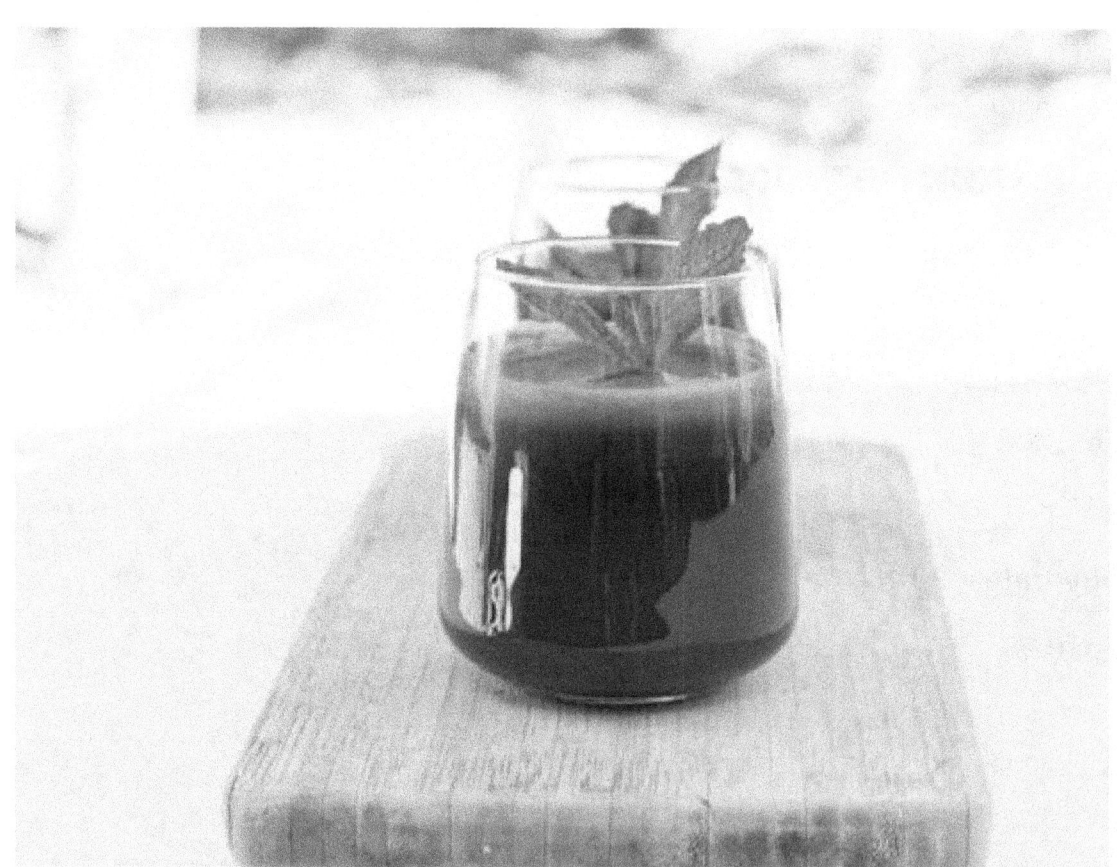

INGREDIENTS

3 carrots

2 apples

2 beetroots

PREPARATION METHOD

1. Wash the ingredients and cut into pieces
2. Pass chunks through juicer
3. Serve chilled

NUTRIENT VALUE PER SERVING

Calories: 321.9

Fat: 1.8g

Carbohydrate: 78.5g

Protein: 5.2g

KALE, GINGER AND PINEAPPLE DETOX DRINK

SERVING SIZE

Serves 4 people

COOKING TIME

5-10 minutes

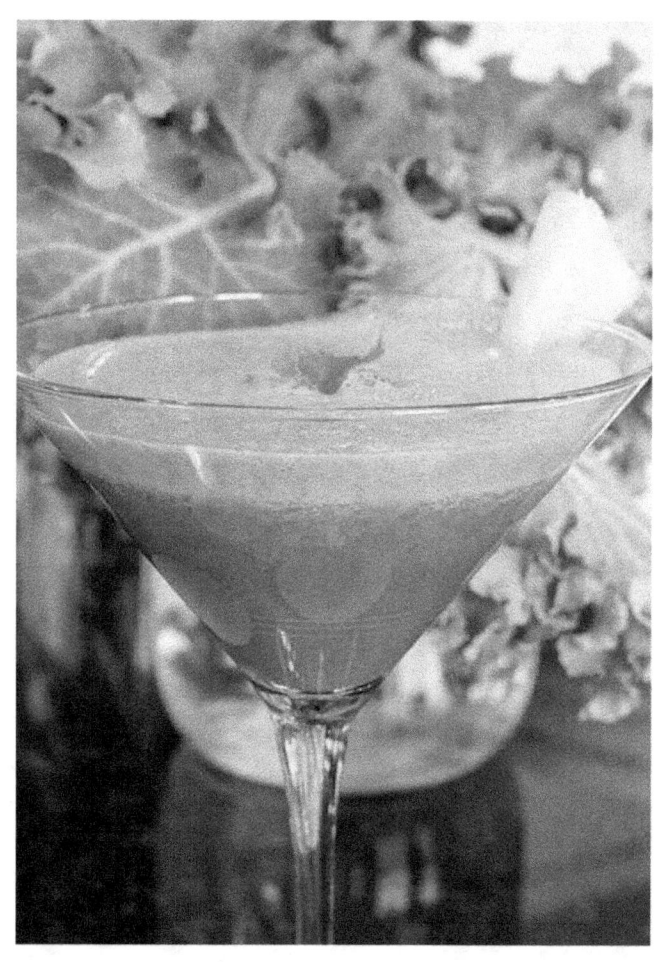

INGREDIENTS

½ cup pineapple

2 cucumbers

4 cups kale

1/8 cup lemon juice

¼ tsp ginger

½ cup mint leaves

PREPARATION METHOD

1. Chop ingredients into pieces
2. Pass through juicer and serve chilled

NUTRIENTS VALUE PER SERVING

Calories: 73

Fat: 0.8g

Carbohydrates: 16.4g

Protein: 3.7g

STRAWBERRY BASIL LIME

SERVING SIZE

1 person

COOKING TIME

5 minutes

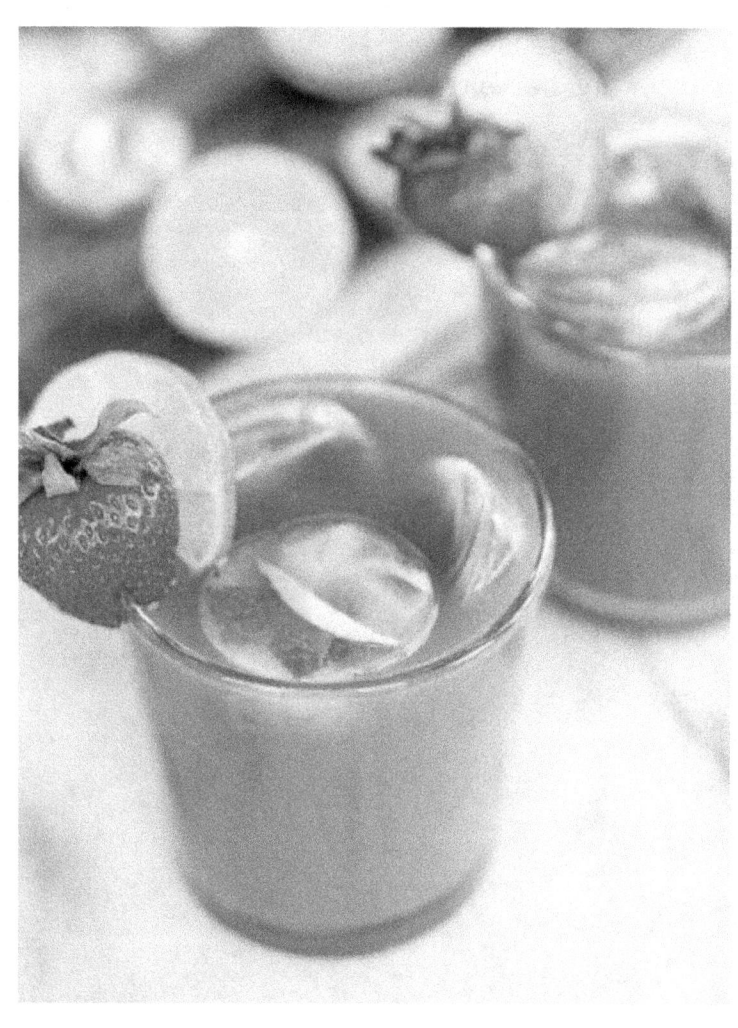

INGREDIENTS

1 cup strawberries

½ cup basil leaves

1 peeled lime

1 cup coconut water

1 tbsp chia seeds

PREPARATION METHOD

1. Blend all the ingredients together
2. Serve chilled

NUTRIENT VALUE PER SERVING

Calories: 167

Fat: 5.1g

Carbohydrates: 33g

Protein: 4.4g

GINGER MINT PINEAPPLE JUICE

SERVING SIZE

1 person

COOKING TIME

5 minutes

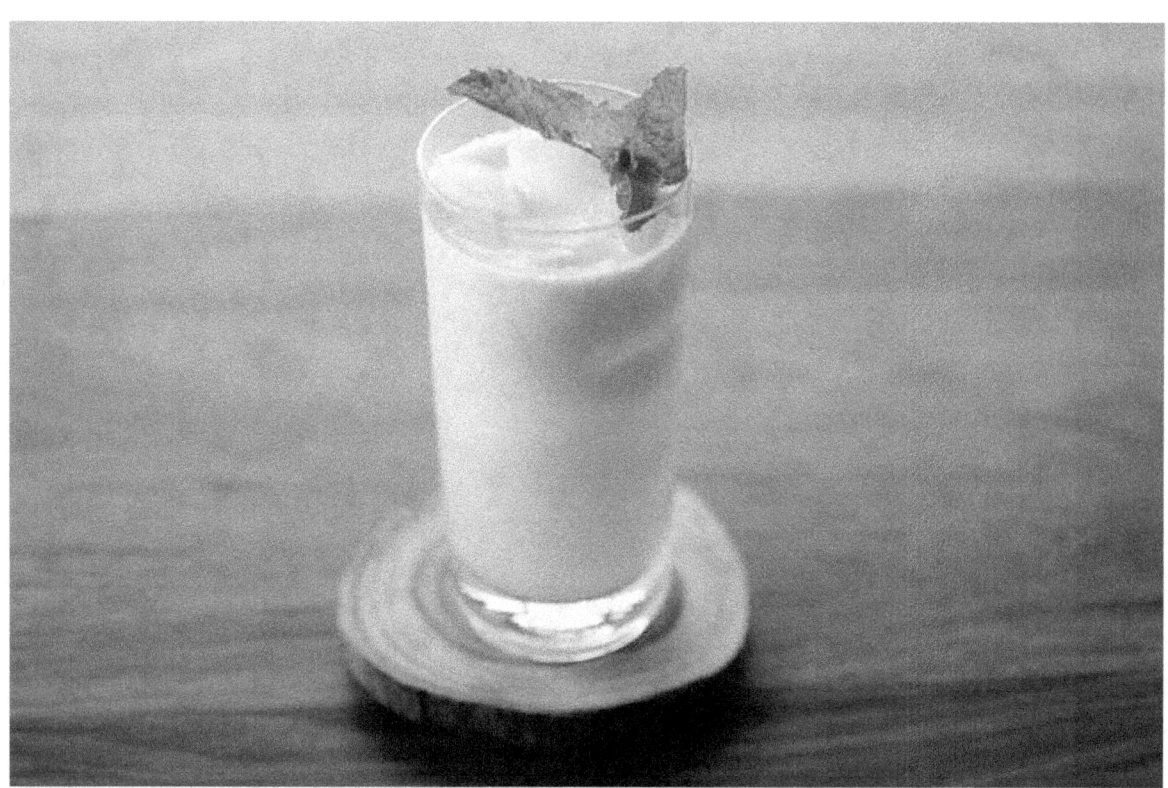

GINGER MINT PINEAPPLE JUICE

INGREDIENTS

¼ cup pineapple

1 piece ginger

½ cup mint leaves

½ cup water

PREPARATION METHOD

1. Blend all the ingredients together and serve chilled.

NUTRIENT VALUE PER SERVING

Calories: 95

Fat: 0.25g

Carbohydrates: 24.9g

Protein: 1.1g

BEETROOT, CARROT AND ORANGE JUICE

SERVING SIZE

1 person

COOKING TIME

5 minutes

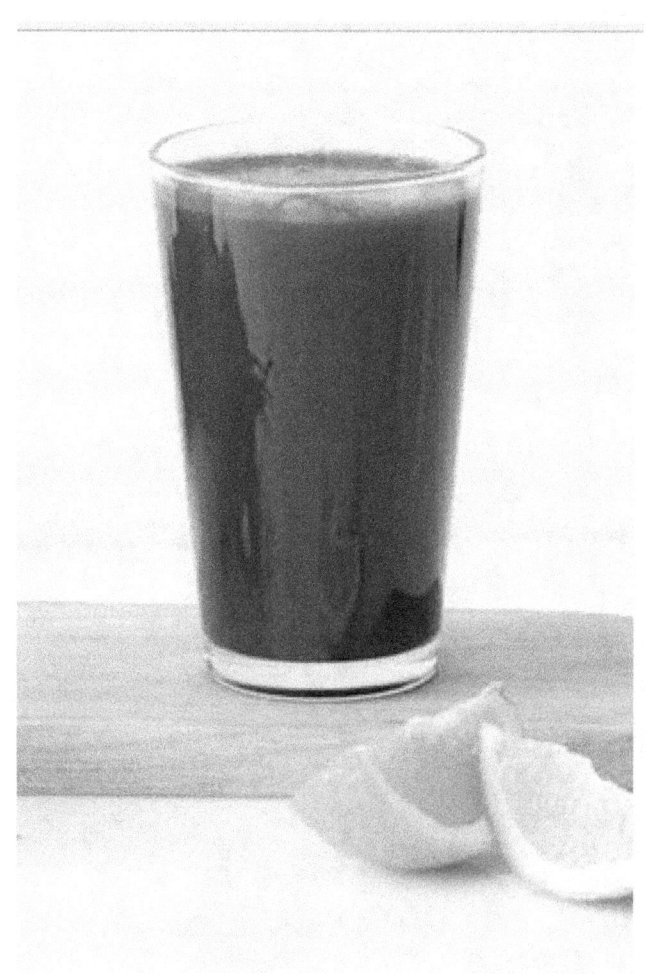

INGREDIENTS

2 oranges

2 carrots

3 beetroots

PREPARATION METHOD

1. Process all the ingredients through a juicer
2. Serve chilled.

NUTRIENT VALUE PER SERVING

Calories: 153

Fat: 0.72

Carbohydrates: 46.2g

Protein: 5.3g

CELERY DETOX

SERVING SIZE

1 person

COOKING TIME

5 minutes

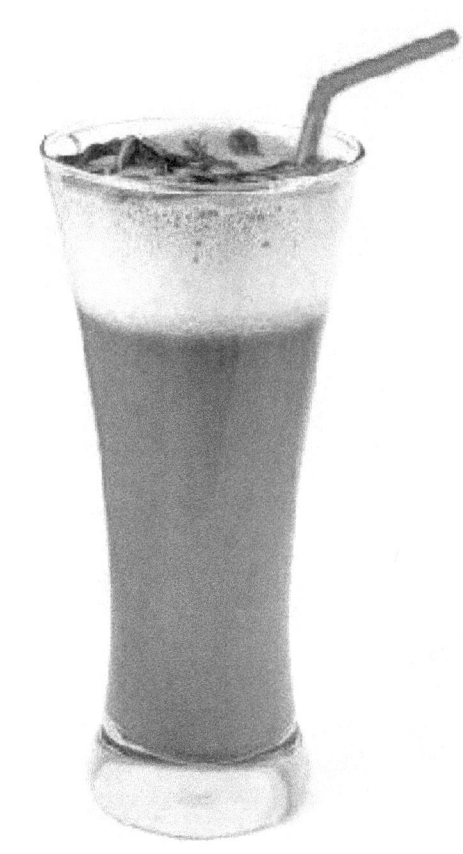

INGREDIENTS

1 apple

½ beetroot

3 carrots

2 large celery

1 handful of parsley

PREPARATION METHOD

1. Process ingredients in a juicer
2. Serve chilled.

NUTRIENT VALUE PER SERVING

Calories: 120

Fat: 0.94g

Carbohydrates: 37.04g

Protein: 3.44g

GOLDEN SPICE

SERVING SIZE

1 person

COOKING TIME

5 minutes

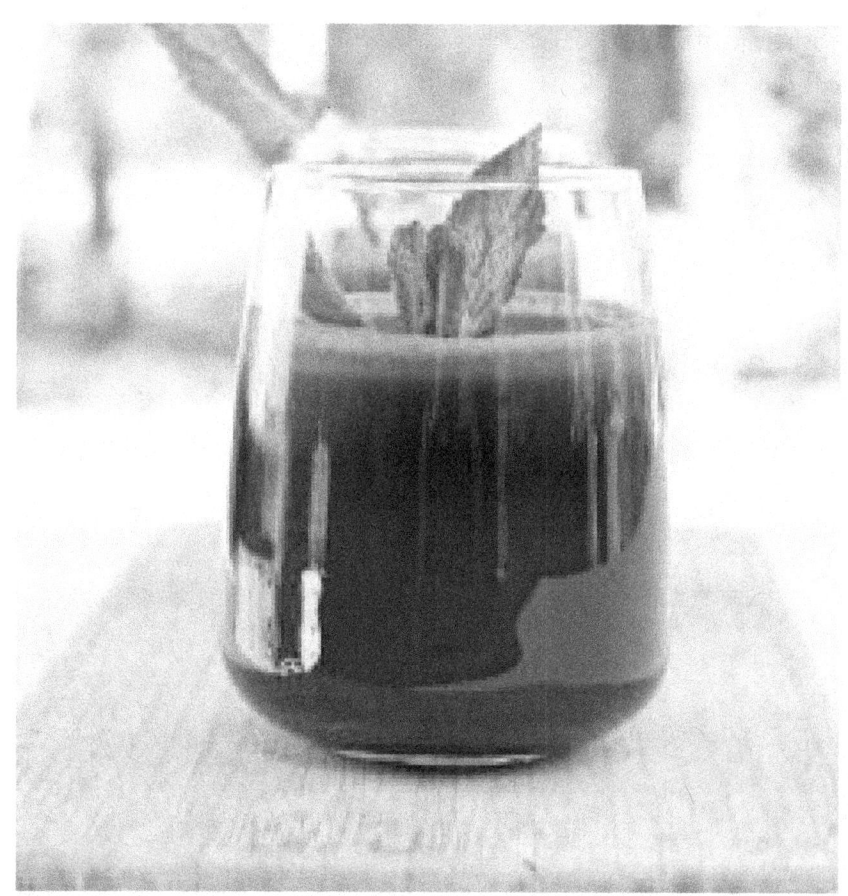

INGREDIENTS

1 apple

1 beetroot

1 ginger

½ lemon

2 slices pineapple

¼ tsp pumpkin pie spice

PREPARATION METHOD

1. Blend all ingredients with water
2. Serve chilled.

NUTRIENT VALUE PER SERVING

Calories: 195

Fat: 0.82

Carbohydrates: 58.65g

Protein: 3.1g

THE LIVER SCRUBBER

SERVING SIZE

1 person

COOKING TIME

5 minutes

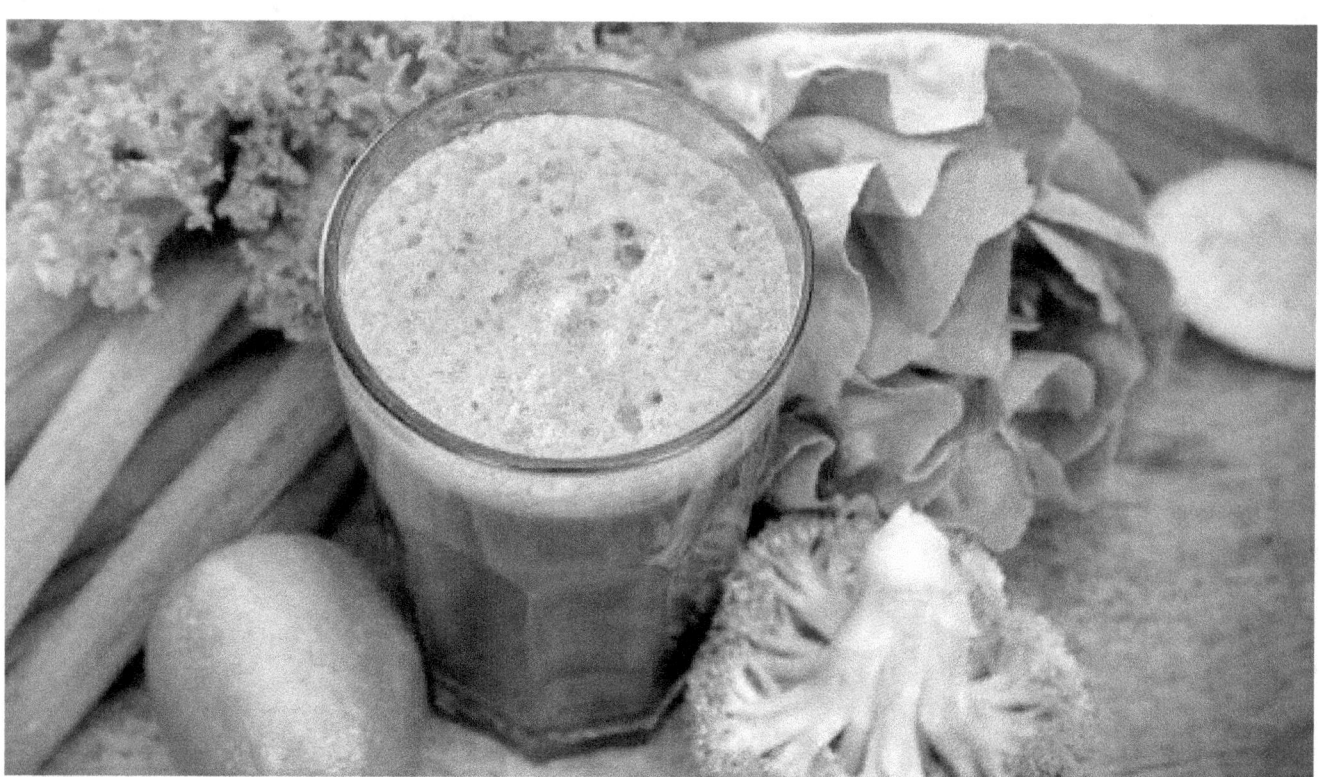

INGREDIENTS

1 apple

1 beetroot

4 carrots

1 large celery

½ ginger

PREPARATION METHOD

1. Process the ingredients in a juicer
2. Stir and serve

NUTRIENT VALUE PER SERVING

Calories: 177

Fat: 1.11g

Carbohydrates: 55.36

Protein: 5.9g

CITRUS BLEND

SERVING SIZE

1 person

COOKING TIME

5 minutes

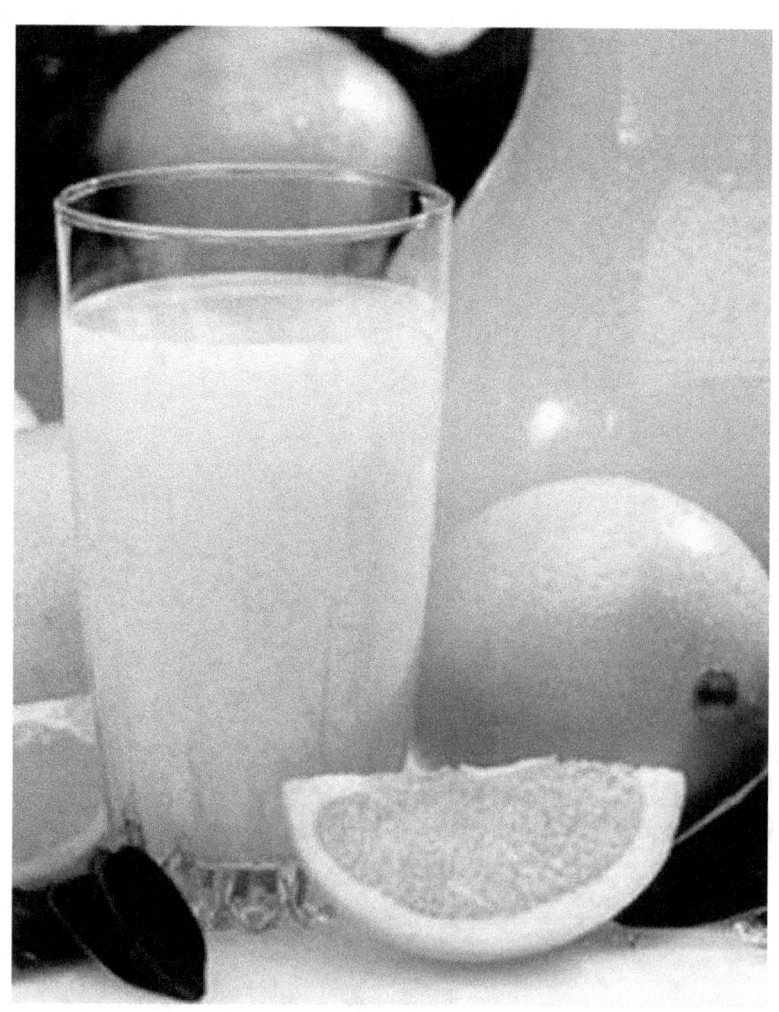

INGREDIENTS

1 lemon

3 oranges

1 grapefruit

1 tsp honey

PREPARATION METHOD

1. Process all ingredients through a juicer
2. Stir and serve

NUTRIENT VALUE PER SERVING

Calories: 96

Fat: 0.2g

Carbohydrates: 22.7g

Protein: 1.2g

CABBAGE JUICE

SERVING SIZE

1 person

COOKING TIME

5 minutes

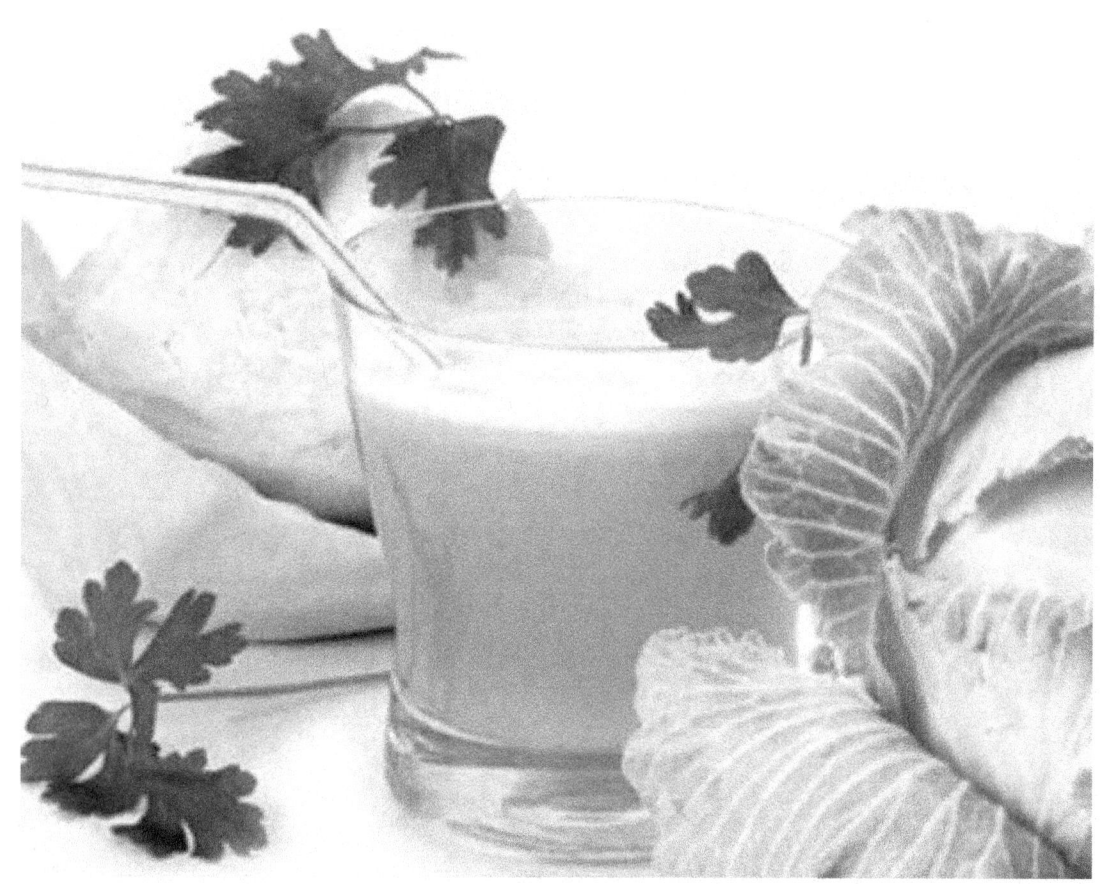

INGREDIENTS

2 pears or carrots

½ cabbage

2 celery sticks

A handful of watercress

PREPARATION METHOD

1. Blend all ingredients together
2. Stir and serve

NUTRIENT VALUE PER SERVING

Calories: 91

Fat: 0.62g

Carbohydrates: 30.7g

Protein: 5.26g

APPLE AND SPINACH JUICE

SERVING SIZE

2 persons

COOKING TIME

5 minutes

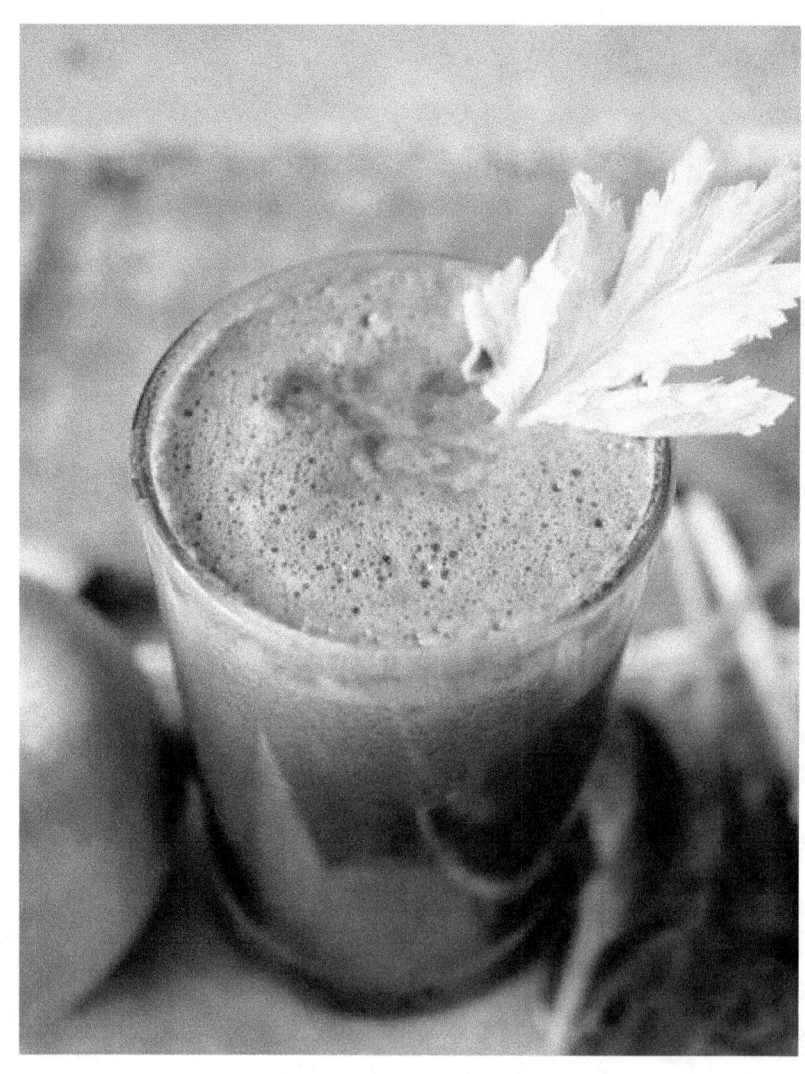

INGREDIENTS

6 cups of spinach

3 green apples

2 handfuls parsley

PREPARATION METHOD

1. Blend all the ingredients together and serve

NUTRIENT VALUE PER SERVING

Calories: 114

Fat: 0.6g

Carbohydrates: 28g

Protein: 2.3g

EXTREME LIVER CLEANSE

SERVING SIZE

1 person

COOKING TIME

5 minutes

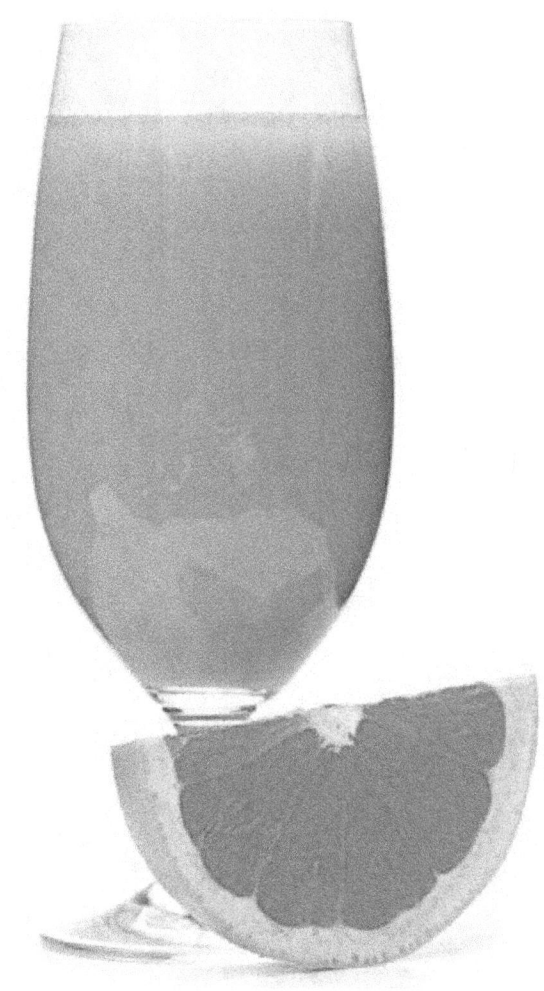

INGREDIENTS

1 grapefruit

½ cup olive oil

3 cups of water

4 tbsp Epsom salt

PREPARATION METHOD

1. Blend all ingredients together, stir and serve.

NUTRIENT VALUE PER SERVING

Calories: 96.3

Fat: 0.25g

Carbohydrates: 22.7g

Protein: 1.2g

FRUIT LIVER CLEANSE

SERVING SIZE

1 person

COOKING TIME

5 minutes

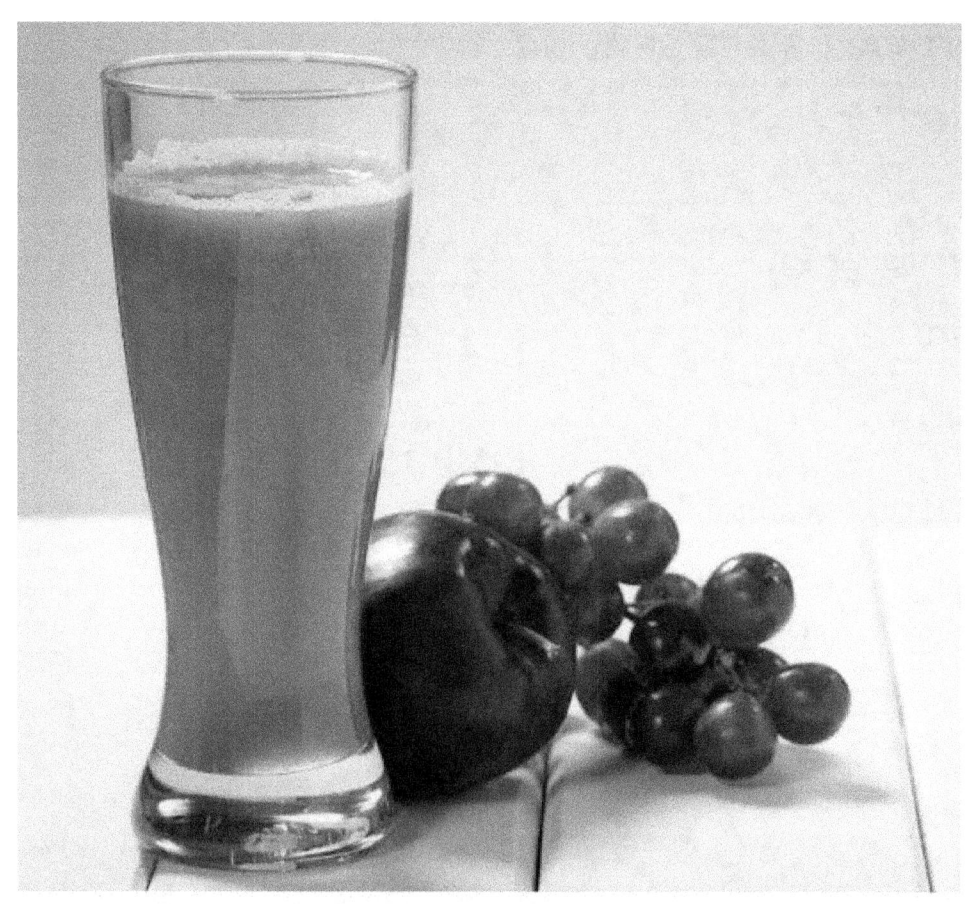

INGREDIENTS

2 apples

A bunch of grapes

½ beetroot

¼ grapefruit

¼ lemon

PREPARATION METHOD

1. Blend all ingredients together, stir and serve.

NUTRIENT VALUE PER SERVING

Calories: 129

Fat: 0.24g

Carbohydrates: 31.7g

Protein: 0.63g

STRAWBERRY AND GRAPE JUICE

SERVING SIZE

1 person

COOKING TIME

5 minutes

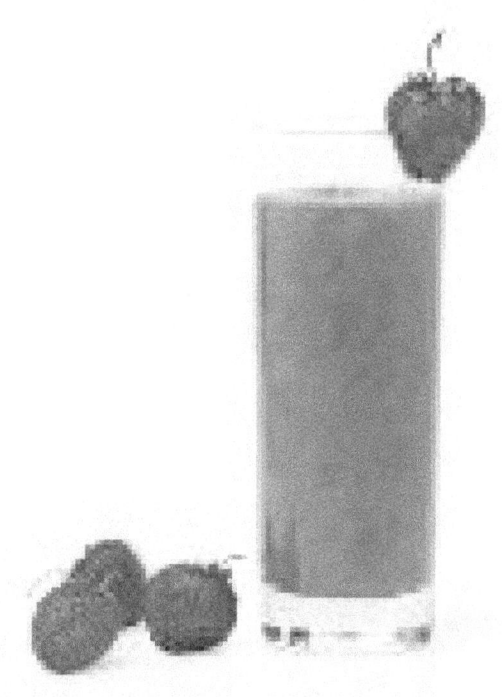

INGREDIENTS

A bunch of grapes

1 cup strawberries

3 apples

Fresh mint

Water

PREPARATION METHOD

1. Blend all the ingredients together
2. Stir and serve

NUTRIENT VALUE PER SERVING

Calories: 110

Fat: 1.42g

Carbohydrates: 18.49g

Protein: 0.71g

PINEAPPLE DETOX JUICE

SERVING SIZE

1 person

COOKING TIME

5 minutes

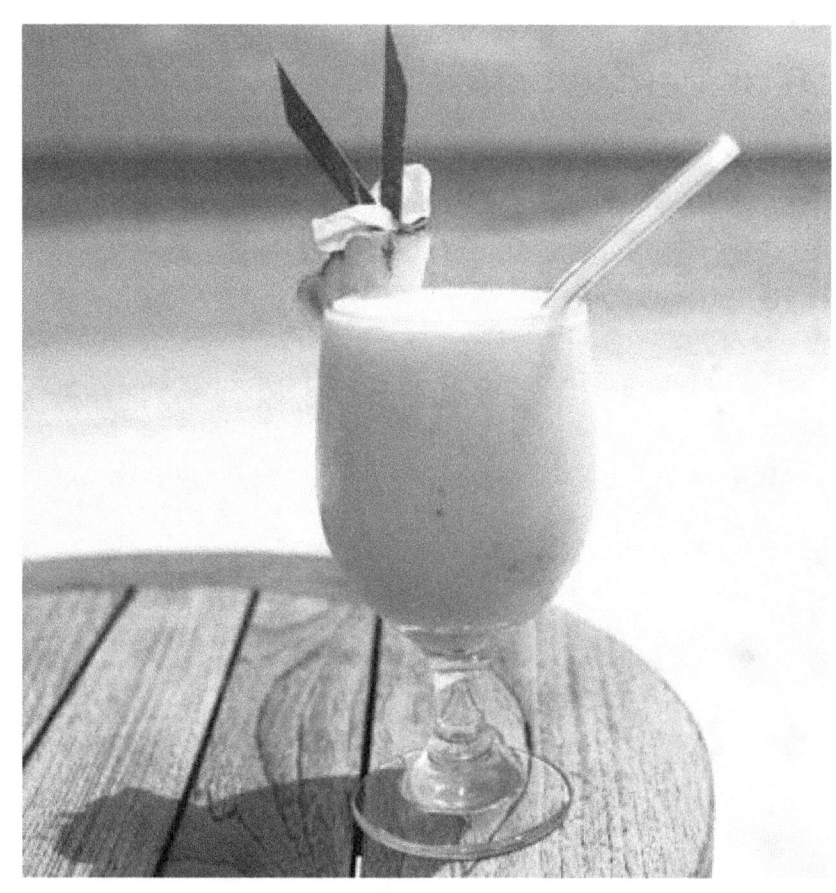

INGREDIENTS

3 slices pineapple

½ cucumber

1/3 cup aloe vera juice

½ cup coconut water

PREPARATION METHOD

1. Blend all ingredients together
2. Serve chilled

NUTRIENT VALUE PER SERVING

Calories: 132

Fat: 0.3g

Carbohydrates: 32.18g

Protein: 0.9g

TURMERIC TEA

SERVING SIZE

1 person

COOKING TIME

10-12 minutes

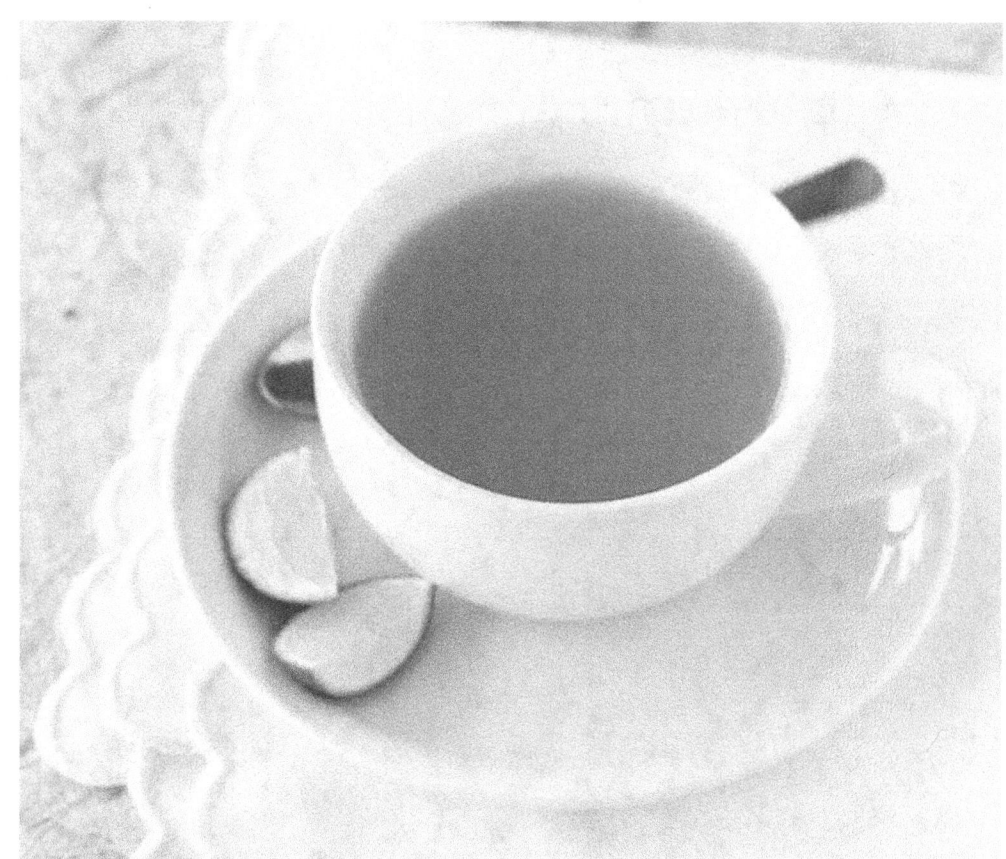

INGREDIENTS

Pinch of nutmeg

Pinch of clove

1 teaspoon cinnamon

1 teaspoon fresh ginger

Turmeric (to taste)

1-2 cups water

Honey

Milk

PREPARATION METHOD

1. Brew the herbs and water together for 10 minutes, after that strain out the herbs and add honey and milk

Alternate method:

2. Add boiled water into blender with spices and blend until smooth. Strain out the tea and milk and honey to taste.

NUTRITIONAL VALUE PER SERVING

Calories: 14g

Fat: 9.88 g

Carbohydrate: 0 mg

Protein: 7.83 g

DETOX DANDELION TEA

SERVING SIZE

2 to 4 persons

COOKING TIME

10-12 minutes

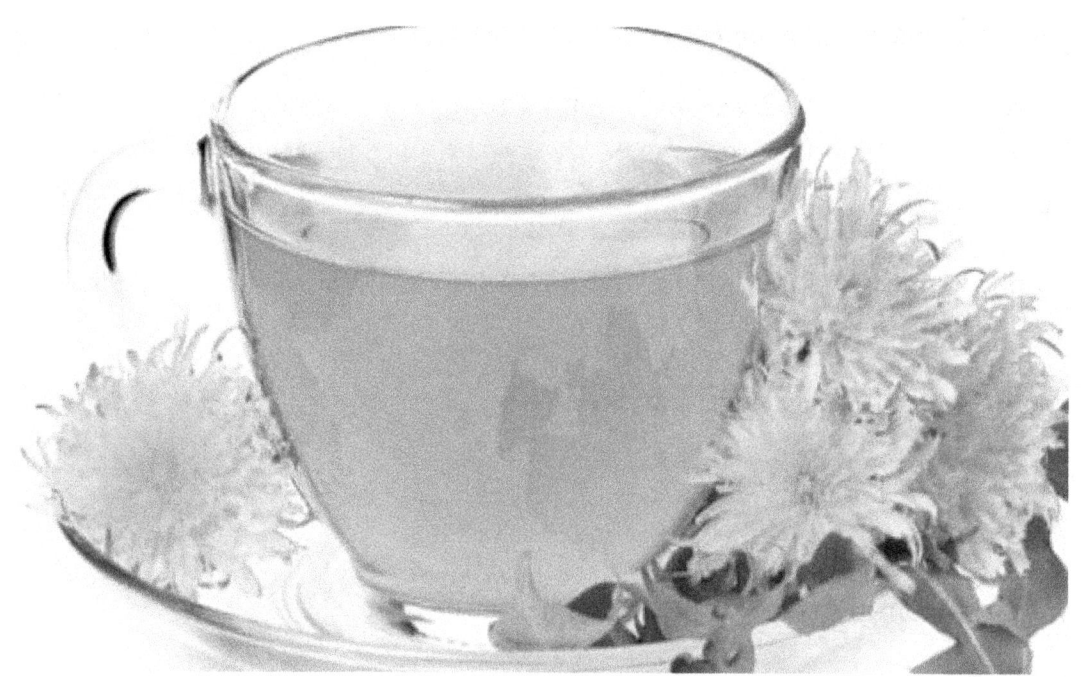

INGREDIENTS

1 tablespoon of dried dandelion roots

2 cinnamon sticks

5-6 pods of cardamom (crushed)

1 teaspoon whole cloves

1 thinly sliced piece of ginger

4 cups boiled water

PREPARATION METHOD

1. Put the dandelion roots and spices in a pot with water
2. Bring to a boil, reduce heat and let it simmer for 10 minutes.
3. Strain the tea in mugs
4. It is ready to serve with milk of your choice and honey to sweeten it a bit.

NUTRIENT VALUE PER SERVING

Calories: 13g

Fat: 0g

Carbohydrate: 3g

Protein: 1g

Detox Lunch Recipes

STEAMED BASS WITH FENNEL, PARSLEY AND CAPERS

SERVING SIZE

2 persons

COOKING TIME

15-20 minutes

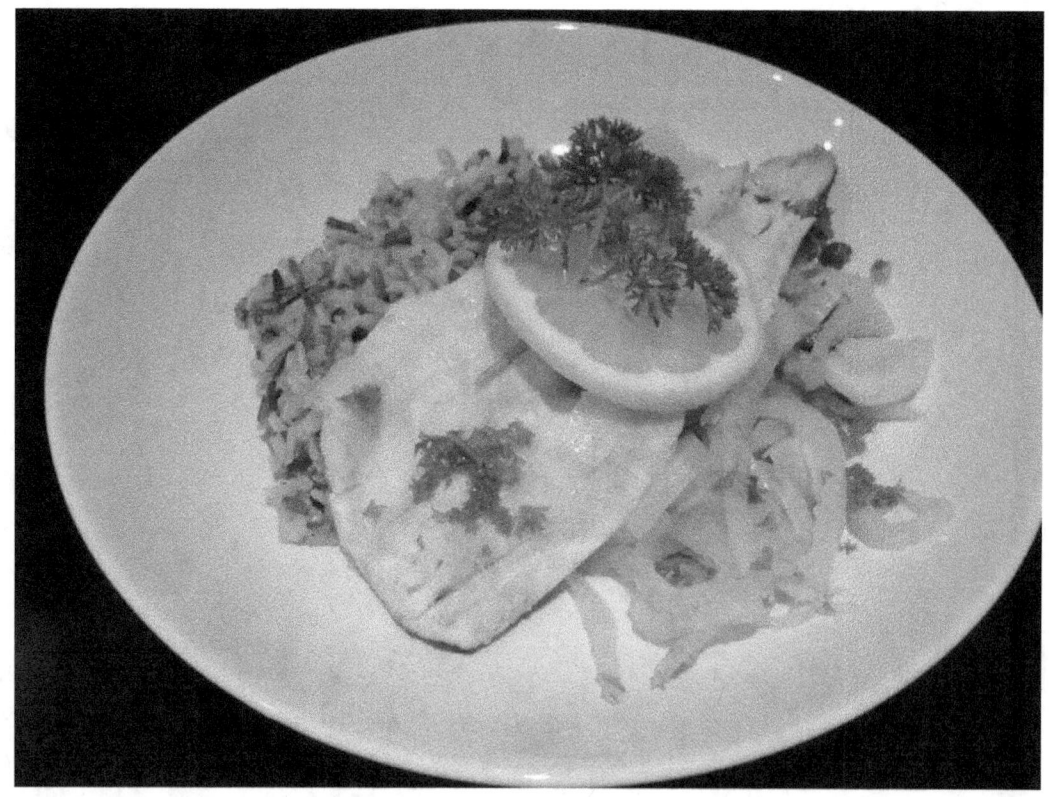

INGREDIENTS

¼ medium sized white onions (sliced)

1 thinly sliced fennel bulb

½ juiced lemon

2/5 ounces of striped bass

½ teaspoon sea salt

1 tablespoon rinsed capers

¼ cup chopped Italian parsley

2 tablespoon extra virgin olive oil

PREPARATION METHOD

1. Take a medium sized saucepan and put onion, fennel and lemon juice. Cover it with approximately 1 inch water
2. When it comes to a boil, simmer for 5 minutes
3. Put 2 portion of fish, seasoned with sea salt after removing from heat
4. Sprinkle with parsley and capers, cover the pan
5. Simmer again for 8-10 minutes until fish is almost flaky
6. Place vegetables in a shallow bowl and put the fish on top. Sprinkle fresh parsley and it is ready to serve.

NUTRITIONAL VALUE PER SERVING

Calories: 427.8

Fat: 16.7g

Carbohydrates: 56.2g

Protein: 15.1g

STIR-FRIED VEGETABLES AND CHICKEN WITH BUCKWHEAT NOODLES

SERVING SIZE

2 persons

COOKING TIME

15-20 minutes

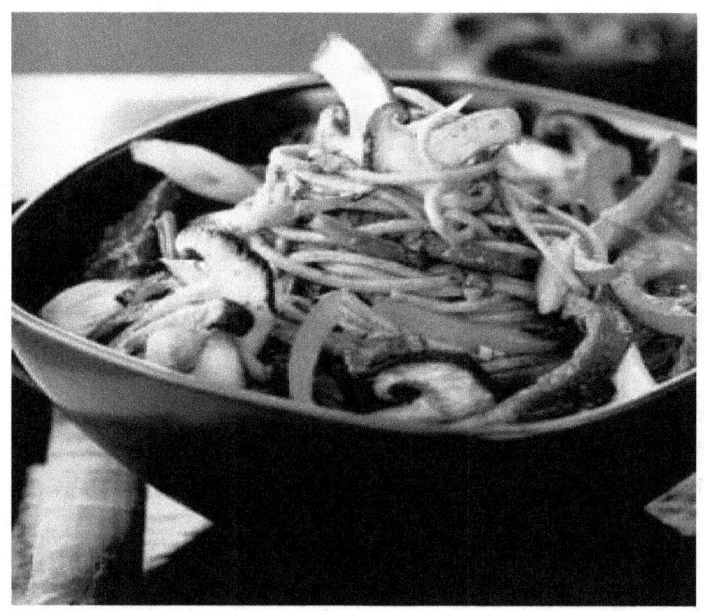

INGREDIENTS

1 packet of buckwheat noodles

1 teaspoon salt

I teaspoon sesame oil

2 garlic cloves

¼ cup sliced ginger

2 thinly sliced carrots

1 cup broccoli florets

1 cup sliced baby bok choy

1 cup sliced zucchini

3 sliced scallions

1 tablespoon nama shoyu or wheat-free tamari

1 cup snap peas

2 grilled and sliced chicken breasts

PREPARATION METHOD

1. Boil 6 cups of water with salt in a large pot
2. Add noodles and boil for further 3 minutes or until tender
3. Drain water and toss noodles in sesame oil lightly and put aside
4. Heat a heavy skillet and add oil, for the stir fry
5. Add garlic and ginger on high heat for one minute, stir with wooden spoon
6. Add the remaining vegetables one at a time except snap peas
7. Use a wooden spoon to toss and flip vegetables
8. Add the nama shoyu and 2 tablespoons of water
9. Add the snap peas finally
10. Toss in a bowl with the noodles and it is ready to serve
11. You can garnish it with fresh cilantro and serve it with chicken breasts on the side

NUTRITIONAL VALUE PER SERVING

Calories: 489.1

Fat: 5.8g

Carbohydrates: 45.1g

Protein: 65.8g

QUINOA SALAD WITH TOASTED ALMONDS

SERVING SIZE

2 persons

COOKING TIME

35 minutes

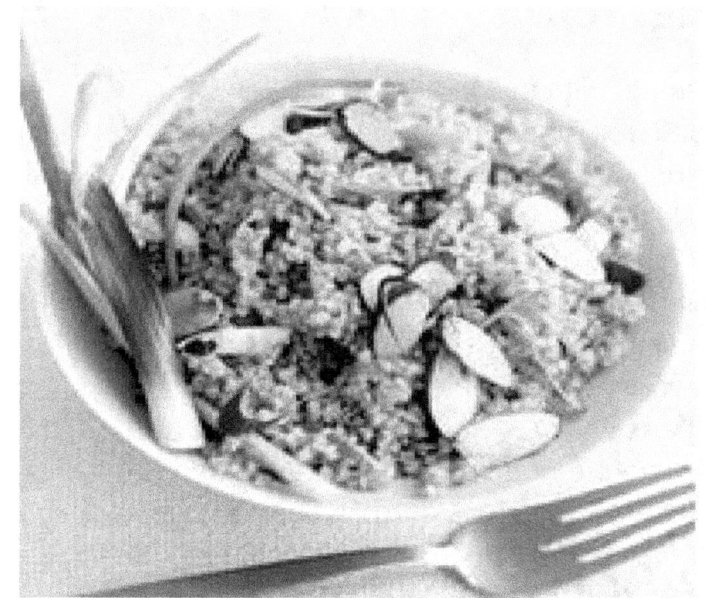

INGREDIENTS

¼ cup almonds

½ cup quinoa

4 teaspoons olive oil

1 yellow bell pepper, cut into chunks of half

2 minced garlic cloves

2 thinly sliced scallions

1/8 teaspoon red pepper flakes

1 teaspoon freshly chopped thyme

¼ teaspoon salt

1 medium zucchini

1 large celery stalk

1 lime

PREPARATION METHOD

1. Toast almonds in preheated oven at 350 degrees, for about 7 minutes until crisp and lightly browned. Set them aside. Rinse quinoa under cold water until the water runs clear and drain well.
2. Heat two teaspoons of olive oil on medium heat in a saucepan. Add yellow pepper, garlic, scallions and red-pepper flakes and cook for 5 minutes until pepper is crisp tender.
3. Stir quinoa, thyme, 1 cup water and ¼ teaspoon salt now and bring to boil. Reduce to a simmer, cover and cook for about 7 minutes. Stir in zucchini, cover and cook again until quinoa is tender, it will take 5-8 minutes. Remove the pan from heat.
4. Stir in celery, almonds, 2 teaspoon oil, and salt. Cool at room temperature and refrigerate. Squeeze lime when ready to eat, if desired.

NUTRITIONAL VALUE PER SERVING

Calories: 268

Protein: 11g

Fat: 19g

Carbohydrates: 44

TOMATO AND BEAN SALAD WITH GRILLED TUNA

SERVING SIZE

4 persons

COOKING TIME

15 minutes

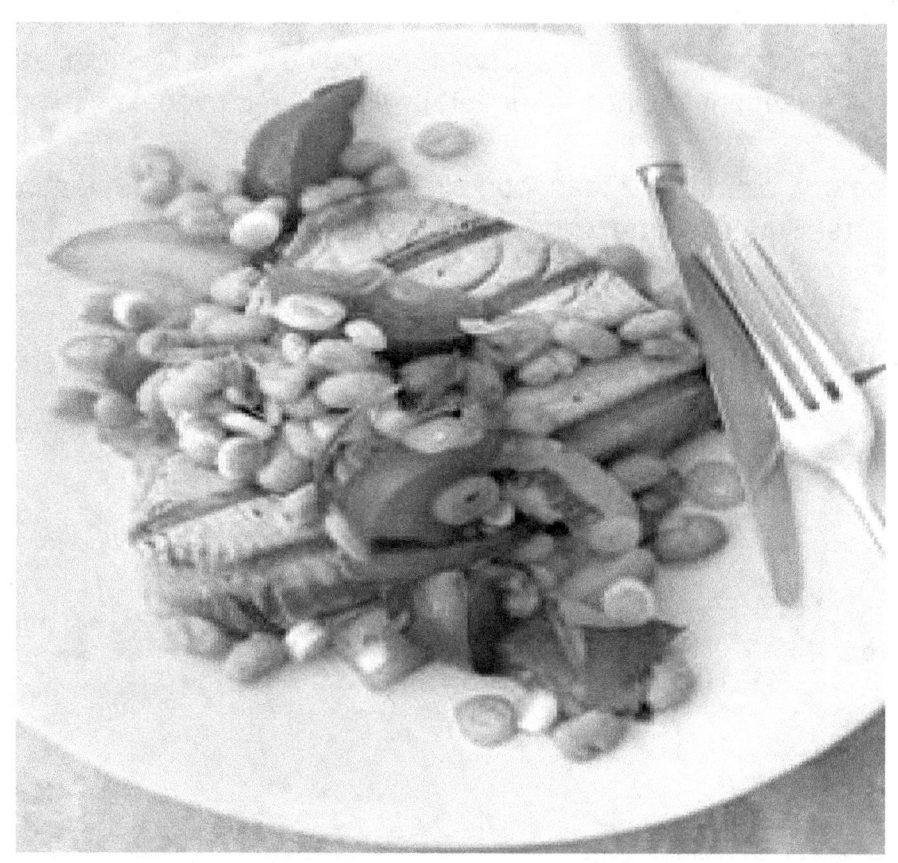

INGREDIENTS

2 tomatoes

1 can of beans, drained and rinsed

¼ cup tarragon leaves

1 tablespoon fresh lemon juice

3 thinly sliced scallions

1 tablespoon olive oil

Salt and ground pepper

4 tuna steaks

PREPARATION METHOD

1. Add tomatoes, beans, tarragon, lemon juice, scallions and oil together and season with salt and pepper, set aside.
2. Heat the grill on medium flame and lightly brush the grates with oil. Season the tuna with salt and pepper on both sides. Grill, until medium rare, turning once, about 2-4 minutes. Tuna can be served with tomato and bean salad.

NUTRITIONAL VALUE PER SERVING

Calories: 305

Fat: 6g

Carbohydrates: 37g

Protein: 27g

DETOX TERIYAKI CHICKEN

SERVING SIZE

1 person

COOKING TIME

20 minutes

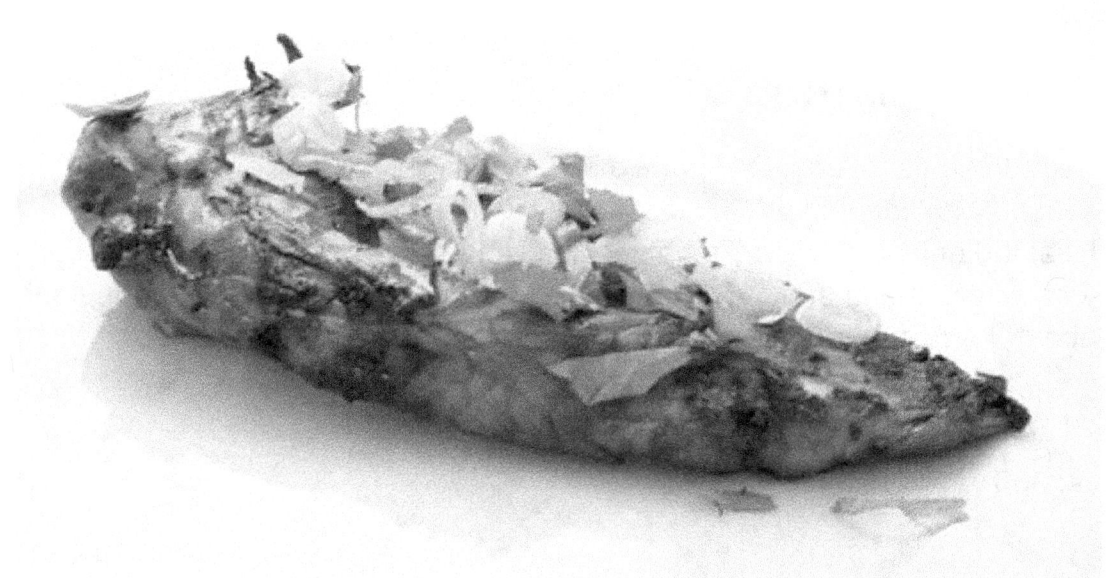

INGREDIENTS FOR SAUCE

1/3 cup balsamic vinegar

1/3 cup agave syrup

1 teaspoon ginger (freshly grated)

¼ teaspoon black pepper

1 teaspoon barley miso

1 teaspoon mirin

1 tablespoon water

INGREDIENTS FOR CHICKEN

I chicken breast

1 finely chopped scallion

4 roughly chopped sprigs cilantro

PREPARATION METHOD

1. To prepare the sauce: Take a small saucepan and combine balsamic, agave, ginger and pepper. Bring to boil, lower down to a simmer and cook for ten minutes. Let it cool and then add miso, mirin and water.
2. Marinate the chicken for at least one hour-up to overnight in the sauce
3. Heat grill on medium heat and grill the chicken for 3-4 on each side or until cooked. Serve with cilantro and scallions.

NUTRITIONAL VALUE PER SERVING

Calories: 671

Fat: 6.7g

Carbohydrates: 96g

Protein: 54.7g

VEGETABLE BROTH SOUP

SERVING SIZE

5 person

COOKING TIME

1 hour and 15 minutes

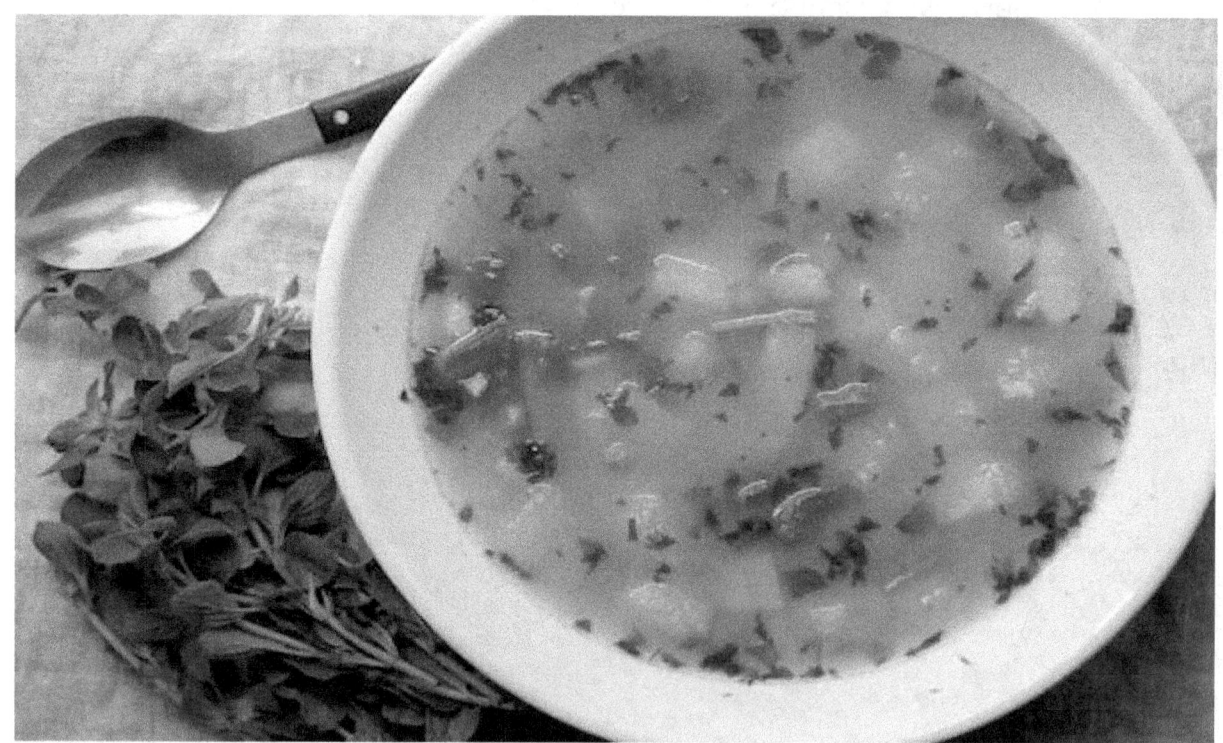

INGREDIENTS

2 roughly chopped red onions

2 roughly chopped stalks celery

1 roughly chopped fennel bulb

2 tsp caraway seeds

2 tsp sea salt

Pepper to taste

1 cup sliced shitake caps

2 chopped large garlic cloves

1 roughly chopped cabbage

2 tbsp paprika

2 quarts water

2 tablespoon chopped oregano

8 sprigs parsley

½ cup chopped parsley

PREPARATION METHOD

1. Combine all ingredients in a pot, except chopped parsley and add 2 quarts of water
2. Bring to a boil and reduce to a simmer, cover for about 1 hour.
3. It is ready to serve, topped with chopped parsley.

NUTRITIONAL VALUE PER SERVING

Calories: 34

Fat: 0g

Carbohydrates: 5g

Protein: 1.5g

FIESTA SLAW

SERVING SIZE

2 person

COOKING TIME

15-20 minutes

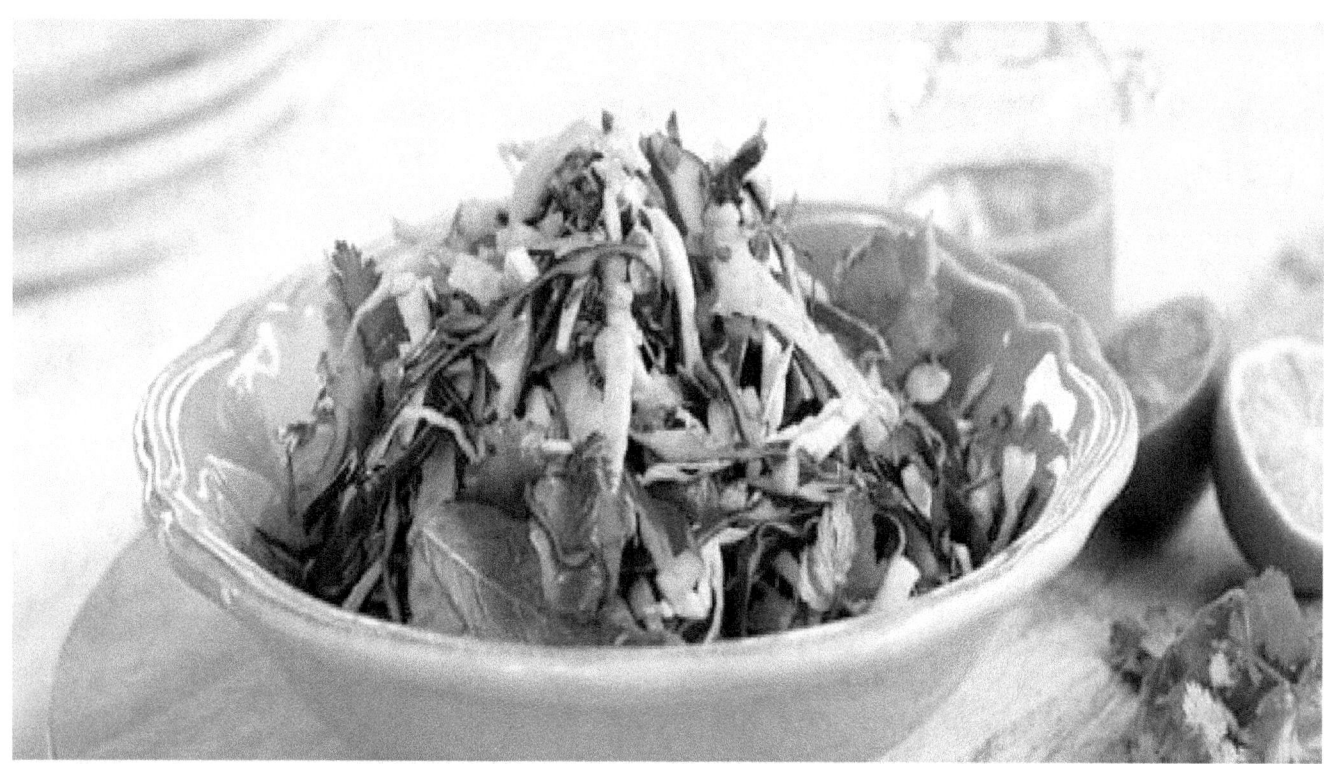

INGREDIENTS

1 large cabbage

2 large carrots

2 sweet red peppers

1 small beet

½ lb raisins

½ bunch cilantro

1 hot pepper

1 piece of fresh ginger

1 meyer lemon

PREPARATION METHOD

1. Grate the cabbage, carrots, beet, sweet peppers, and hot pepper using your food processor or a hand grater.
2. Chop the cilantro and dice the fresh ginger.
3. Juice it up with lemon
4. Mix all the ingredients in a large bowl and let it sit for 20 minutes.

NUTRIENT VALUE PER SERVING

Calories: 249

Fat: 12g

Carbohydrates: 8.4g

Protein: 3.7g

LETTUCE LEAF WRAPS

SERVING SIZE

Makes 8 rolls

COOKING TIME

10-15 minutes

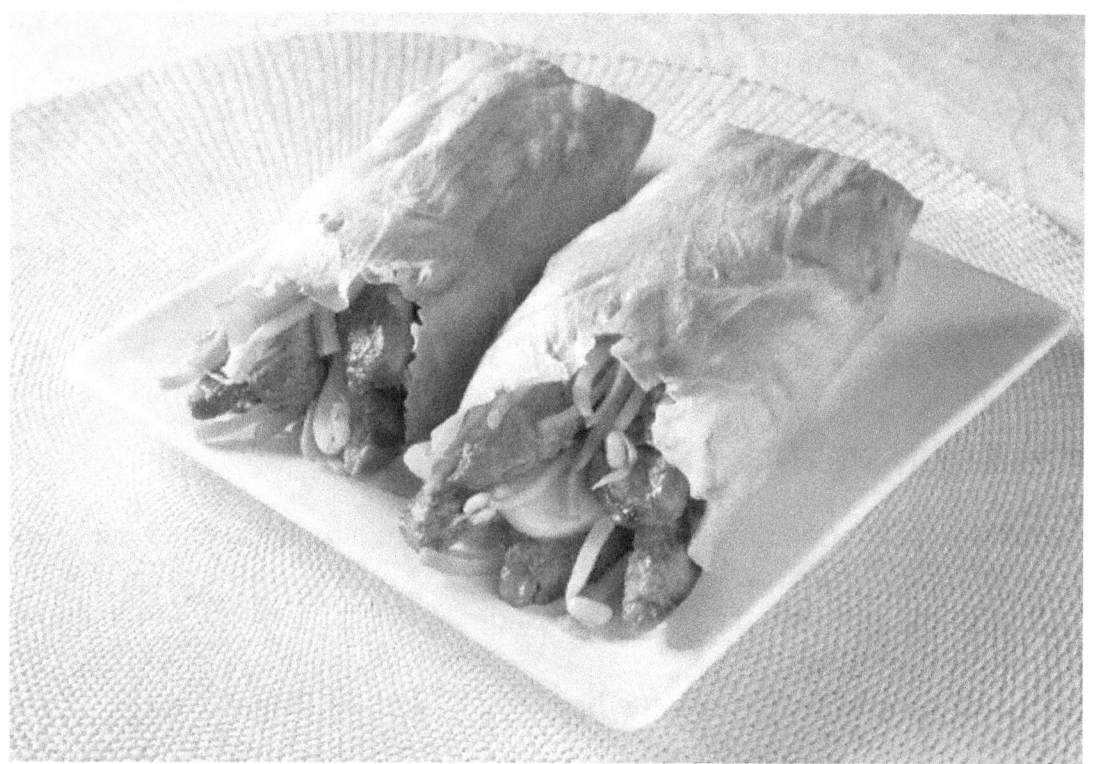

INGREDIENTS

8 large lettuce leaves

1 cup guacamole

1 cup grated carrot

½ horizontally cut cucumber (sliced into pieces)

1 cup sprouts

1 cooked chicken breast (shredded)

PREPARATION METHOD

1. Wash and dry the lettuce leaves and cut the bottom 1 inch of stem
2. Put 2 tablespoons of guacamole on the lettuce leaf. Spread it across the leaf carefully, so as not to tear it
3. Spread 2 tablespoons of carrot, cucumber and sprouts over the guacamole
4. Lay 2 tablespoons of chicken on the vegetables and roll up the lettuce leaf like a burrito.
5. The wrap is complete and ready to serve.

NUTRIENT VALUE PER SERVING

Calories: 250

Fat: 4g

Carbohydrate: 31g

Protein: 22g

BREAKFAST PATTIES

SERVING SIZE

Makes 12 patties

COOKING TIME

20-30 minutes

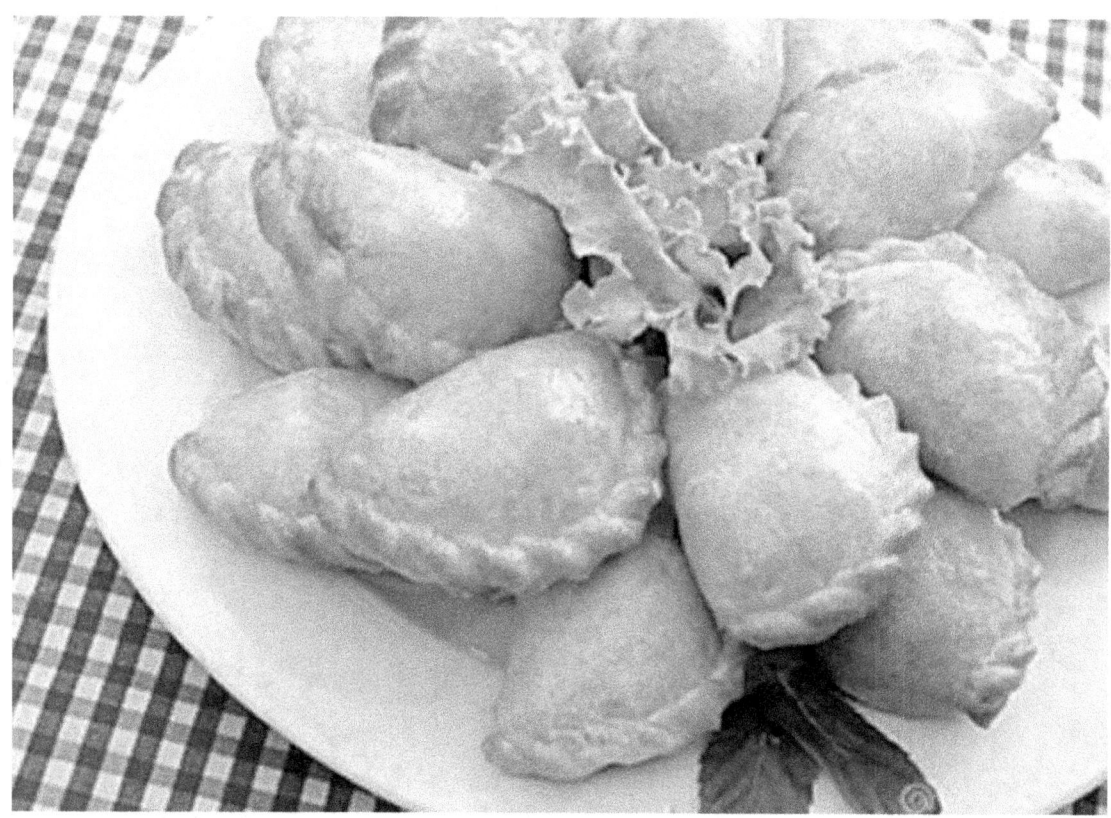

INGREDIENTS

2 tablespoons olive oil

2 tablespoons brown rice or spelt flour

1 tablespoon soy sauce

1 ½ cup warm vegetable stock

1 cup rolled oats

½ cup chopped yellow onion

½ teaspoon dried sage

½ teaspoon dried thyme

1cup chopped raw nuts

1 cup cooked brown rice

1 cup minced shiitake or button mushrooms

PREPARATION METHOD:

1. Add oil, flour and soy sauce in a large skillet over medium-low heat. Whisk well for the ingredients to combine
2. Whisk in vegetable stock and cook until it thickens, whisk more until 2 minutes
3. Add oats, onion, sage, thyme, nuts, rice and mushrooms after removing from heat. Combine the ingredients well by stirring and transfer the contents to a medium mixing bowl.
4. Allow the mixture to set at room temperature for 10 minutes. Refrigerate until cool, for about 20 minutes
5. Preheat oven to 350 degree F. line a baking sheet with parchment paper
6. Take the mixture from refrigerator and scoop ¼ cup into a patty. Place on the baking sheet and continue until done.
7. Bake for 20 minutes and it should be ready to serve.

NUTRIENTS VALUE PER SERVING

Calories: 180

Fat: 16g

Carbohydrates: 23g

Protein: 5g

POACHED APPLES WITH VANILLA YOGURT

SERVING SIZE

Serves 4

COOKING TIME

55 minutes

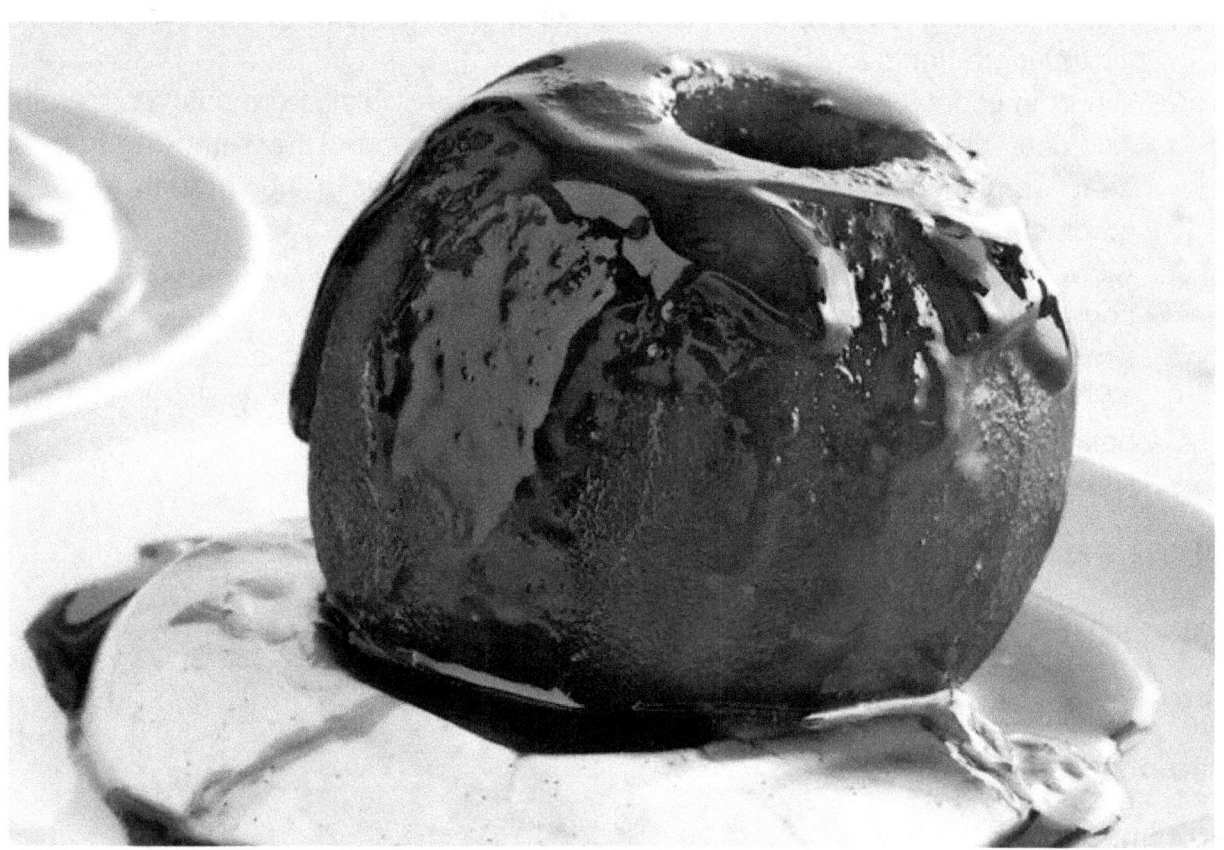

INGREDIENTS

1 ½ cup red wine

¾ cup sugar

1/3 cup orange juice

2 orange peel strips

1 lemon peel strip

1 cinnamon stick

1 whole star anise

4 apples

1 cup yogurt

1 ½ tbsp honey

1 vanilla bean

PREPARATION METHOD

1. Boil wine, sugar, orange juice, orange peel, lemon peel, cinnamon stick and star anise in 2 cups water. Add apples and rotate apples occasionally until tender.
2. Set apples aside in a plate. Strain the liquid in a saucepan. Heat the liquid until syrupy and reduce it to ¾ cup.
3. Blend the yogurt, honey and vanilla seeds in a small bowl until smooth.
4. Divide yogurt sauce among servings, place apples on top and serve with drizzled sauce.

NUTRIENT VALUE PER SERVING

Calories: 322.9 Kcal

Fat: 1.4g

Carbohydrates: 73.9g

Protein: 5.3g

RAW CHOCOLATE PUDDING

SERVING SIZE

Makes 2 ½ cups

COOKING TIME

5-10 minutes

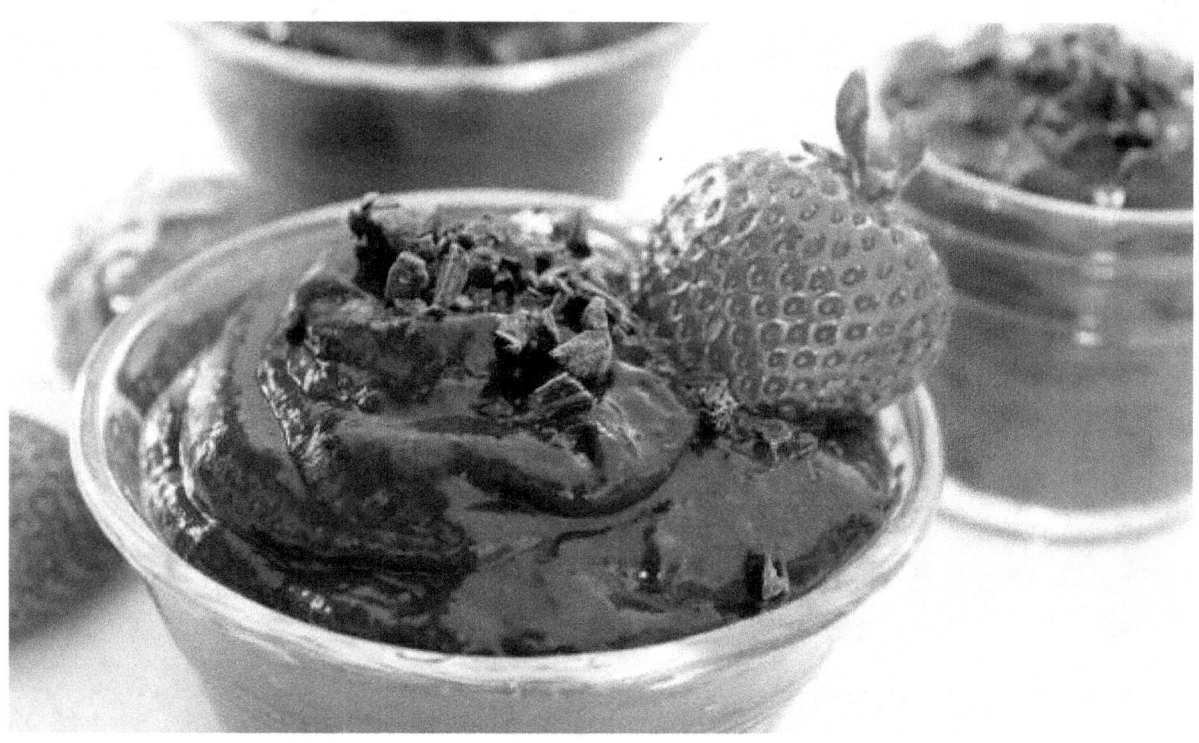

INGREDIENTS

10 fresh dates (cut in quarter)

10 dried figs without stem

2 tablespoons unsweetened cocoa powder

2 tablespoons raw nut butter

1 teaspoon vanilla extract

1 ½ - 2 cups filtered water

PREPARATION METHOD

1. Put the dates, figs, cocoa, nut butter, vanilla extract in blender with 1 cup of water and blend until fruits break down
2. Add water for consistency and blend until a smooth and creamy mixture is made
3. Serve with a cherry on top

NUTRIENT VALUE PER SERVING

Calories: 737

Fat: 13g

Carbohydrates: 168g

Protein: 6g

PESTO RICE

SERVING SIZE

Serves 2 people

COOKING TIME

10-12 minutes

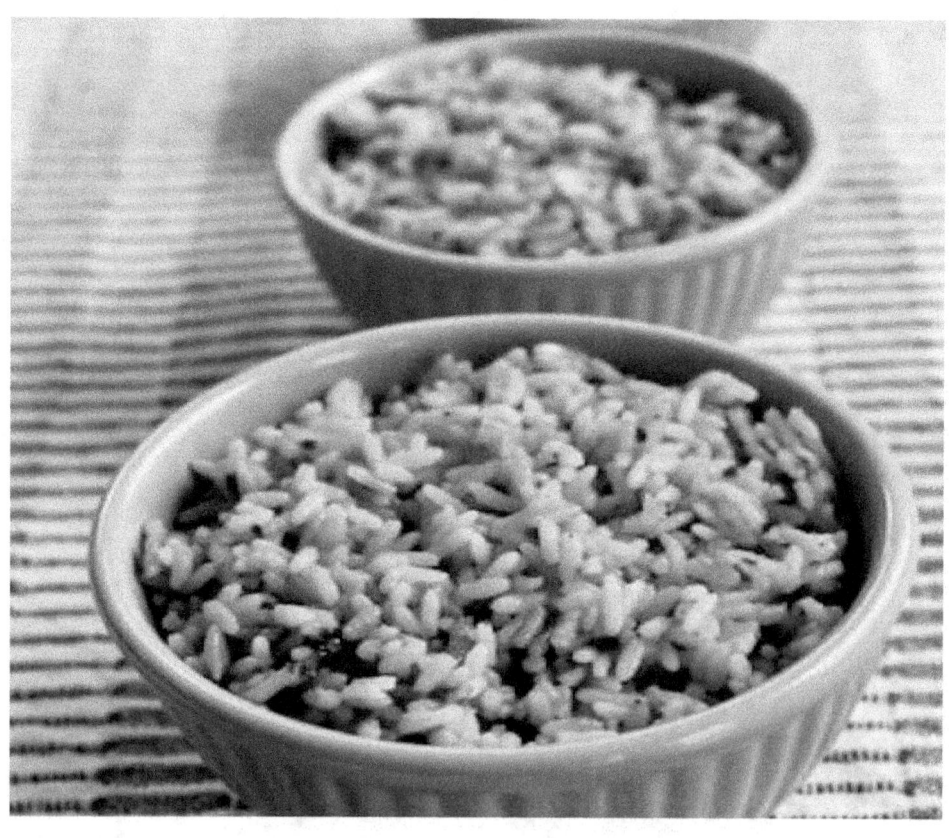

INGREDIENTS

2 tablespoons pesto sauce

1 diced tomatoe

1 oz crumbled feta

2 cup fresh spinach

2 cup cooked brown rice

Salt to taste

Pepper to taste

PREPARATION METHOD

1. Mix all the ingredients in a bowl
2. Put in microwave for 1 minute
3. Ready to serve fresh

NUTRIENT VALUE PER SERVING

Calories: 350.6

Fat: 11.5g

Carbohydrates: 52.6g

Protein: 9.7g

CUCUMBER MINT SOUP

SERVING SIZE

Makes serving for 5-6 persons

COOKING TIME

5-10 minutes

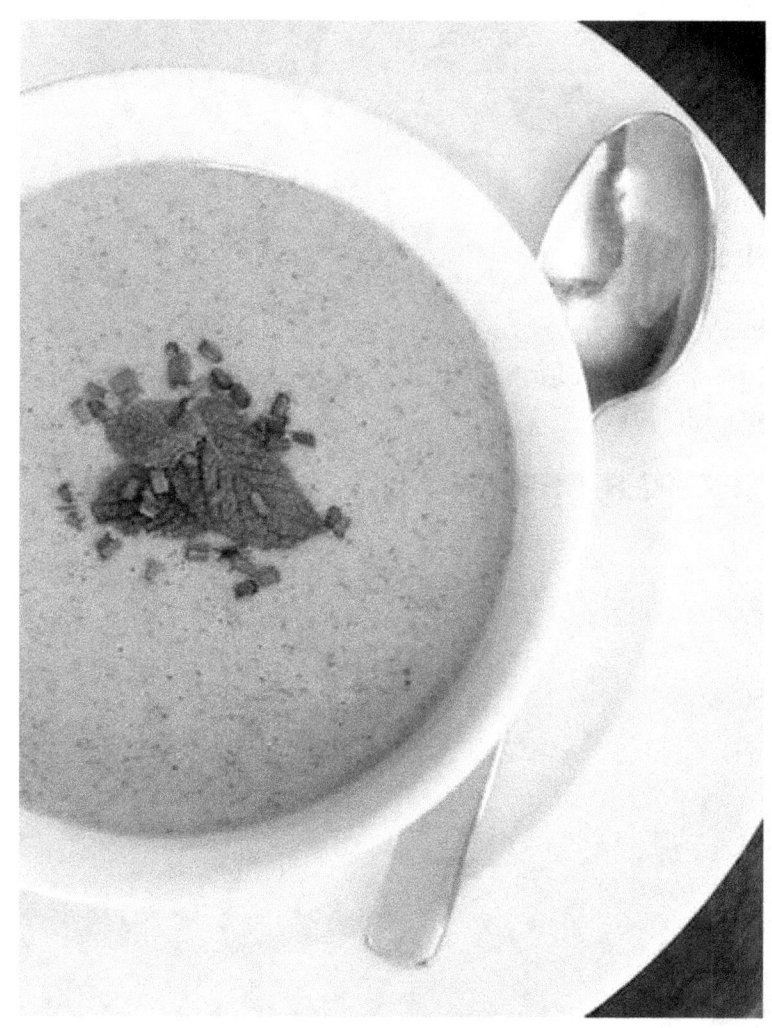

INGREDIENTS

1 ½ pound chopped and peeled cucumbers

1 cup chopped mint

¼ cup chopped chives

2 teaspoons chopped garlic

1 ¼ cup plain nonfat yogurt

½ tablespoon lemon juice

1 teaspoon sea salt

A pinch of black pepper

PREPARATION METHOD

1. Combine cucumber, mint, chives and garlic in a blender and blend until smooth
2. Pour the mixture in a large bowl and mix the remaining ingredients. Stir well.
3. Put in refrigerator for 2-4 hours and serve chill.

NUTRIENT VALUE PER SERVING

Calories: 57

Fat: 0.7g

Carbohydrates: 9.3g

Protein: 3.6g

Dinner recipes

GINGER CARROT SOUP

SERVING SIZE

Served 8 persons

COOKING TIME

30-35 minutes

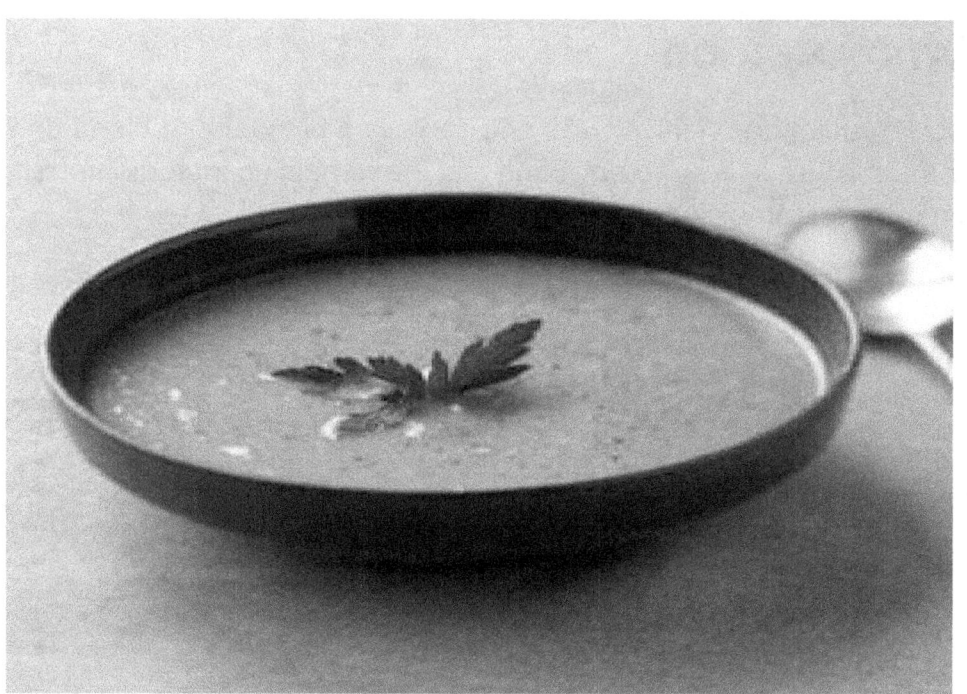

INGREDIENTS

2 tablespoons olive oil

1 cup chopped onions

Kosher salt

1 tablespoon minced garlic

2 tablespoons minced peeled ginger

2 pounds peeled and chopped carrots

1 medium peeled and chopped russet potato

6 cups chicken or vegetable stock

¼ cup pine nuts

1 1/3 low fat yogurt

1 teaspoon honey

1 teaspoon minced fresh thyme

Black pepper

PREPARATION METHOD

1. Combine olive oil and onion in a pot over medium-high heat. Sprinkle ½ teaspoon salt and cook for 10 minutes
2. Add garlic and ginger and cook, careful not to burn the mixture. Add carrots, potato and the chicken or vegetable stock. Cover and cook until carrots and potato are tender. This should take around 20-25 minutes
3. Meanwhile, in a small pan lightly toast the pine nuts over high heat. Set aside to cool
4. Combine yogurt, honey, thyme and pepper in a separate small bowl
5. Puree the soup in batches in blender or use an immersion blender until it is smooth. Serve with the yogurt mixture and pine nuts.

NUTRIENT VALUE PER SERVING

Calories: 262

Fat: 10.8g

Carbohydrates: 31.4g

Protein: 10.2g

RED PEPPER WALNUT RELISH

SERVING SIZE

Makes 1 cup

COOKING TIME

1 hour

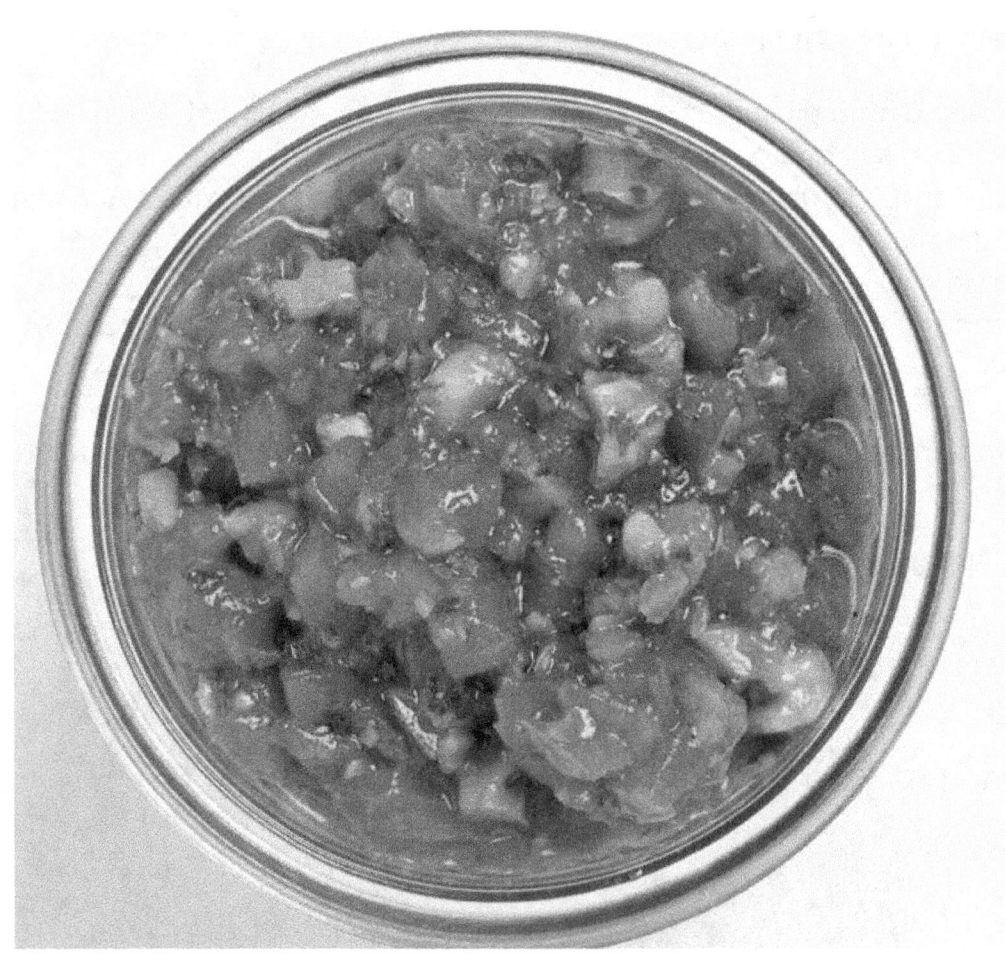

RED PEPPER WALNUT RELISH

INGREDIENTS

¼ cup walnuts

½ tsp balsamic vinegar

½ tsp lemon juice

1 garlic clove

1 tbsp fresh mint

1 tsp pepper

2 red bell peppers

Salt to taste

PREPARATION METHOD

1. Toast walnuts and chop coarsely
2. Broil bell peppers and softened and place in bowl covered with plastic wrap for 15 minutes to steam.
3. In a small bowl, toss bell peppers, garlic, mint, oil, pepper, lemon juice and walnuts. Season with salt and its ready to serve.

NUTRIENT VALUE PER SERVING

Calories: 80 kcal

Fat: 6g

Carbohydrates: 6g

Protein: 3g

SPICED PUMPKIN SEED AND CASHEW CRUNCH

SERVING SIZE

Makes 1 cup

COOKING TIME

35 minutes

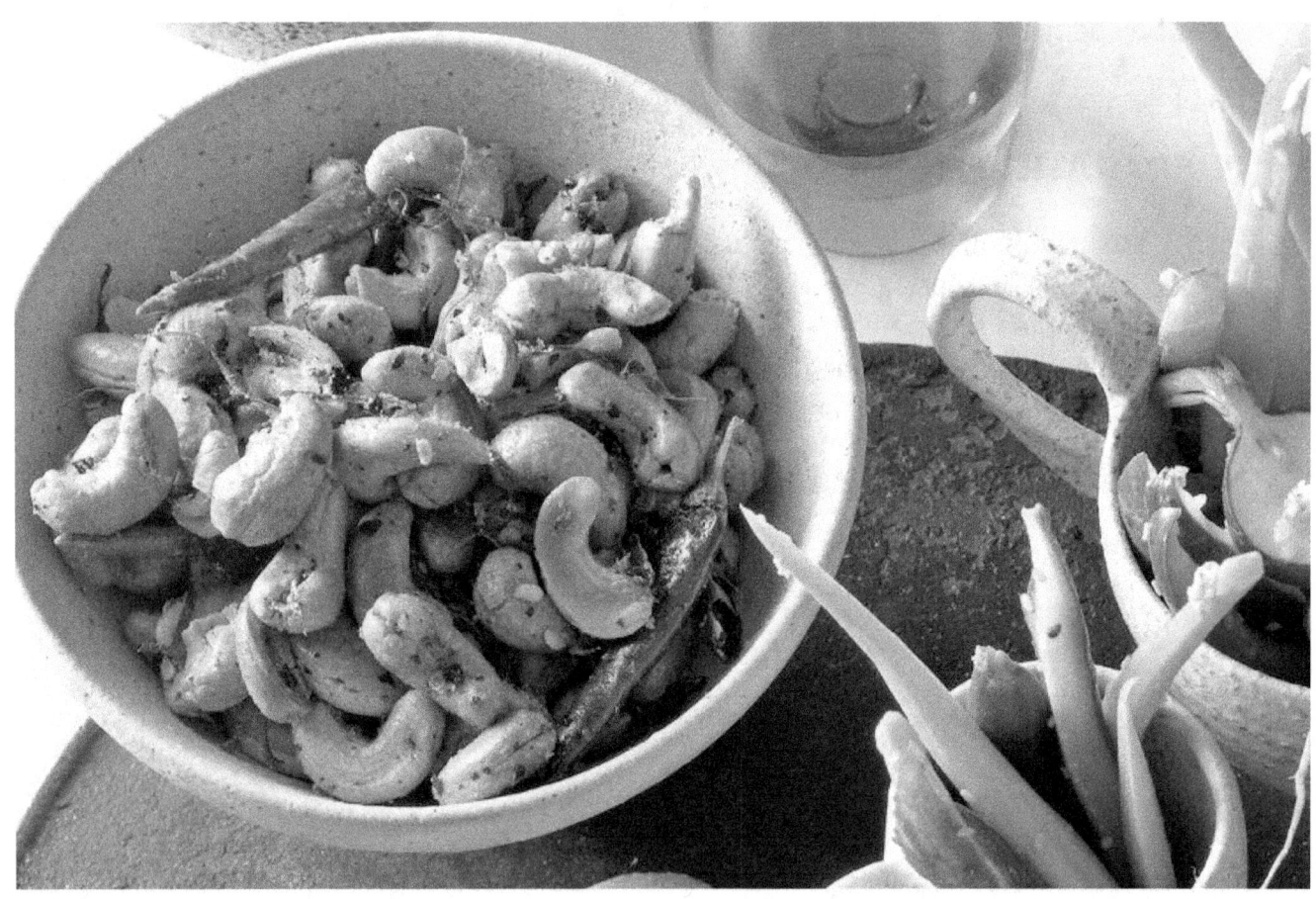

INGREDIENTS

¼ cup pumpkin seeds

¼ cup raw cashews

¼ cup sunflower seeds

½ tsp curry powder

½ tsp kosher salt

1 egg white

1 tsp agave syrup

1/8 tsp cayenne pepper

Vegetable oil spray (nonstick)

PREPARATION METHOD

1. Preheat oven at 300 degrees. Roast nuts and seeds on baking tray coated with oil spray
2. Whisk egg white, agave, curry powder, salt and cayenne in a bowl
3. Bake the mixture once with the seeds, for 20-25 minutes until it is golden brown
4. Let it cool and serve

NUTRIENT VALUE PER SERVING

Calories: 120 Kcal

Fat: 9g

Carbohydrates: 5g

Protein: 1g

KALE AND BRUSSELS SPROUT SALAD

SERVING SIZE

8-10 persons

COOKING TIME

10-15 minutes

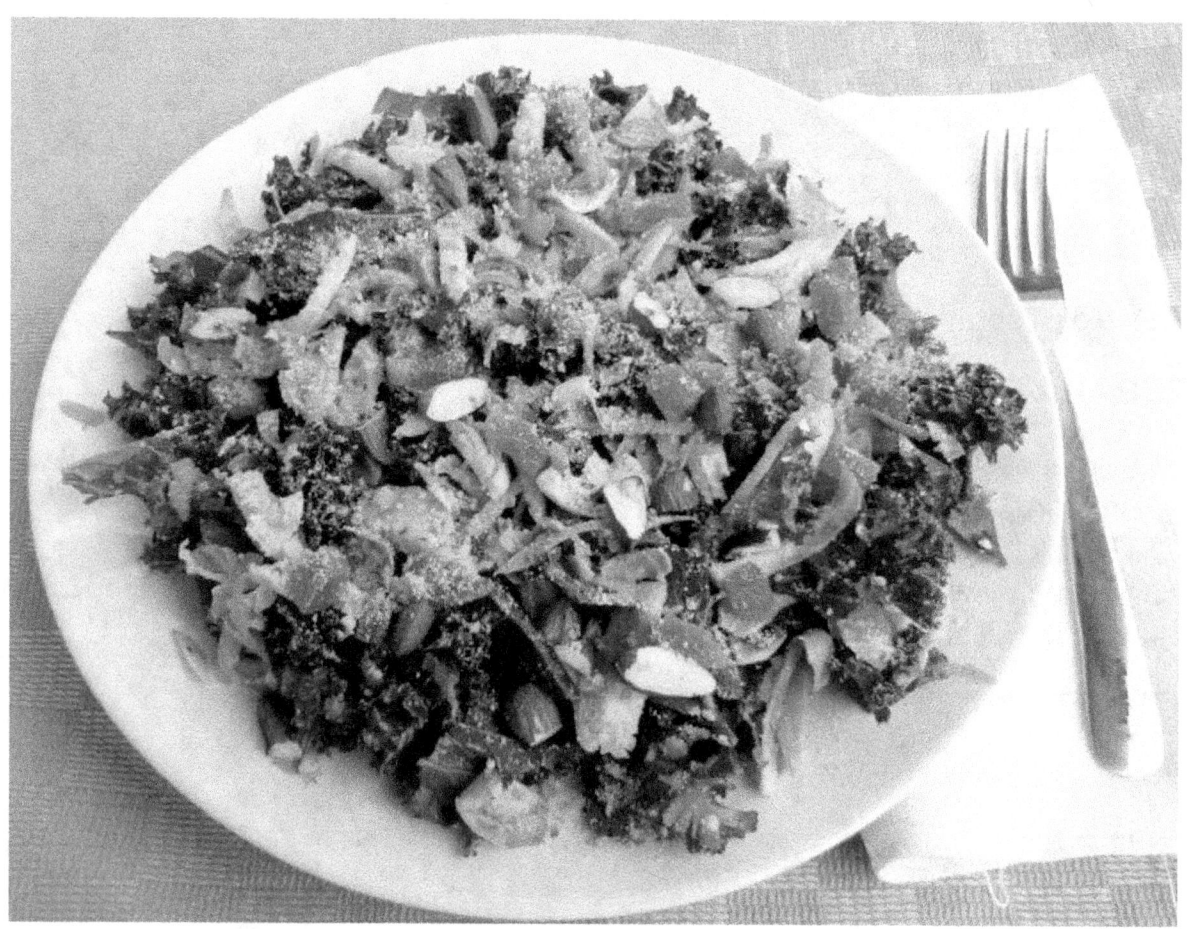

INGREDIENTS

¼ cup lemon juice

¼ tsp kosher salt

½ cup olive oil

1 cup grated Pecorino

1 grated garlic clove

1 tbsp minced shallot

1/3 cup almonds

12 ounces grated Brussels sprouts

2 bunches of Tuscan kale

2 tbsp Dijon mustard

Black pepper to taste

PREPARATION METHOD

1. Mix lemon juice, Dijon mustard, shallot, garlic, salt and pepper in bowl and set aside
2. Heat 1 tbsp oil and stir almonds in until brown.
3. Add olive oil to the lemon juice mixture, stir in almonds and nuts and serve fresh.

NUTRIENT VALUE PER SERVING

Calories: 195.6 Kcal

Fat: 15.3g

Carbohydrates: 8.7g

Protein: 8.1g

SWORDFISH SKEWERS WITH SWEET PEPPER SALAD

SERVING SIZE

1 person

COOKING TIME

30 minutes

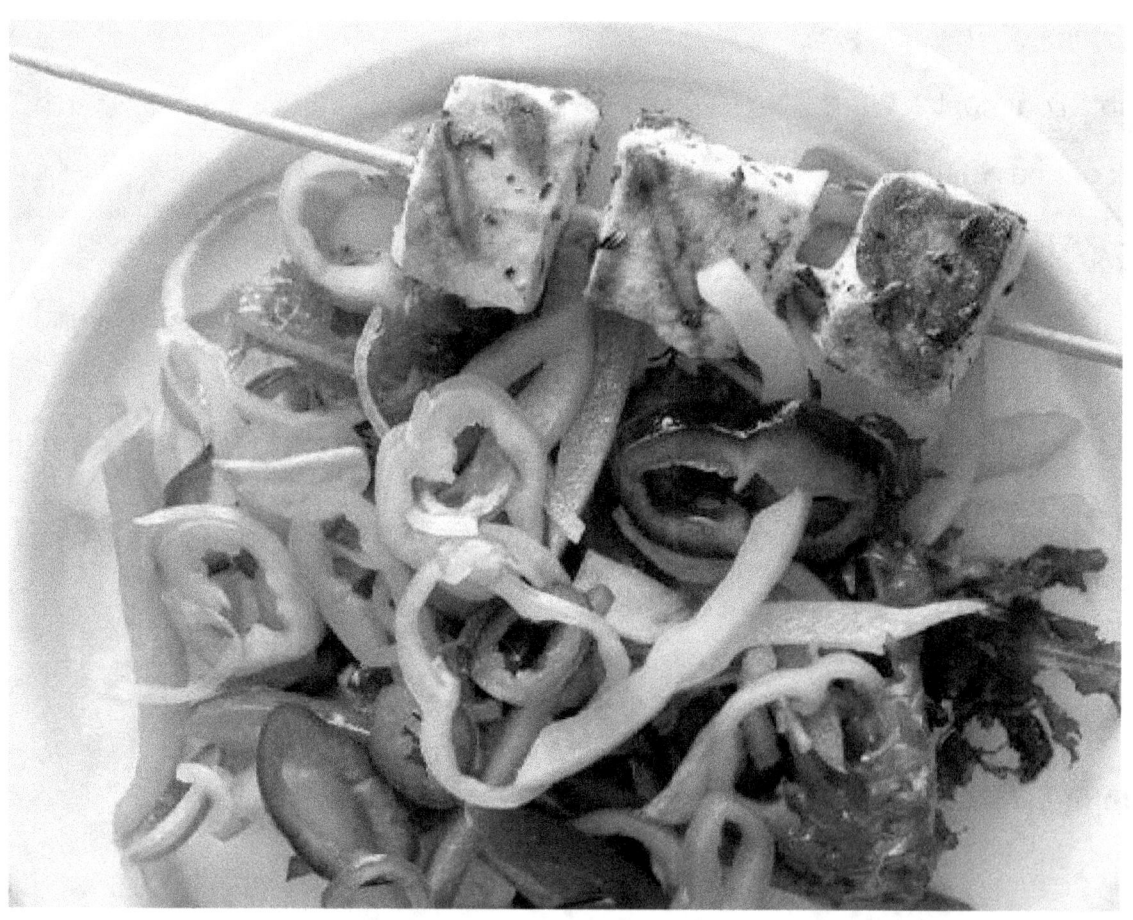

INGREDIENTS

½ onion thinly sliced

1 lemon

1 tbsp fresh rosemary

1 thinly sliced jalapeno

1" thick swordfish steaks cut in cubes

2 tbsp vinegar

3 thinly sliced garlic cloves

4 assorted sweet peppers

4 ounce arugula

7 tbsp olive oil

Salt and pepper to taste

PREPARATION METHOD

1. Heat oil and cook garlic until golden brown. Reserve for garnish
2. In a bowl combine onion, peppers, jalapeno, vinegar, ¼ cup garlic oil and arugula. Season with salt and pepper and let it remain for 10 minutes
3. Place the swordfish cubes on skewer, brush with oil and season with rosemary, salt and pepper. Grill for about 2 minutes on each side until lightly brown.
4. Serve in plates garnished with garlic and lemon.

NUTRIENT VALUE PER SERVING

Calories: 380 Kcal

Fat: 29g

Carbohydrates: 8g

Protein: 23g

POACHED SALMON WITH AVOCADO SAUCE

SERVING SIZE

4 persons

COOKING TIME

20-25 minutes

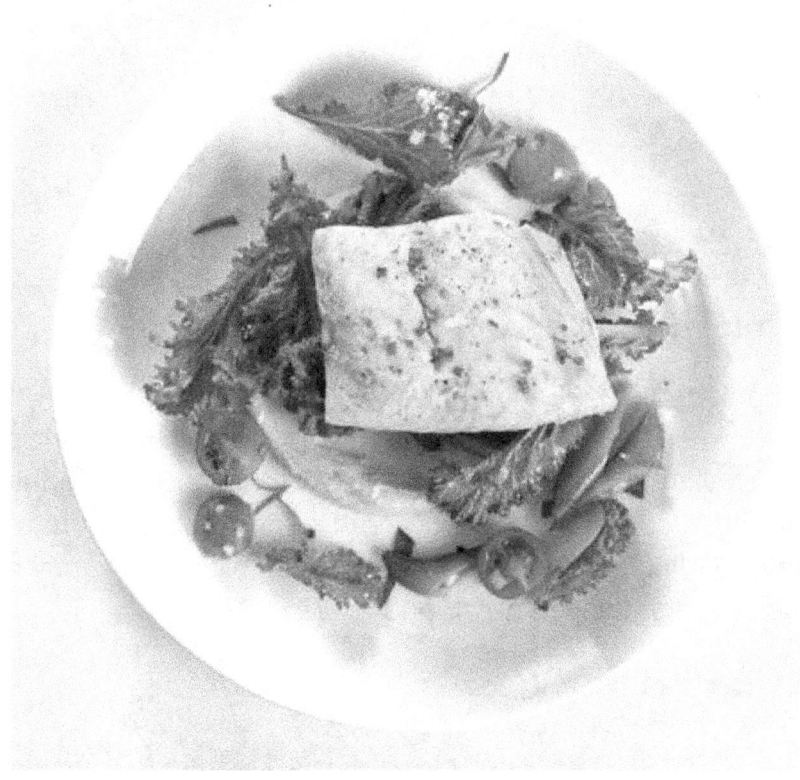

INGREDIENTS

½ tsp cumin

1 cup yogurt

1 tbsp lemon juice

1 tbsp minced shallot

2 cups sugar snap peas

2 halved ripe avocados

2 tbsp chives

2 tbsp olive oil

20 halved cherry tomatoes

20 tarragon leaves

28 ounce skinless salmon fillets

4 cups arugula

4 limes wedges

Pepper and kosher salt

PREPARATION METHOD

1. Season fish with salt, pepper and half of tarragon
2. Bring broth to boil, add salmon and cook for 10-15 minutes until medium rare. Transfer to plate and let it cool
3. Boil salted water and cook sugar snap peas for 2 minutes. Cool the peas in cold water
4. Add 1 tbsp yogurt, lime juice and cumin to avocado in food processor, season with salt and pepper
5. Scoop ½ cup avocado puree in each plate. Mix remaining tarragon, peas, arugula and shallot in bowl, add 1 tbsp oil, lemon juice, salt and pepper. Toss and divide in plates. Top with salmon and serve with lemon wedges.

NUTRIENT VALUE PER SERVING

Calories: 470 Kcal

Fat: 29g

Carbohydrates: 26g

Protein: 31g

HOMEMADE MUESLI

SERVING SIZE

Makes 4 cups

COOKING TIME

10 minutes

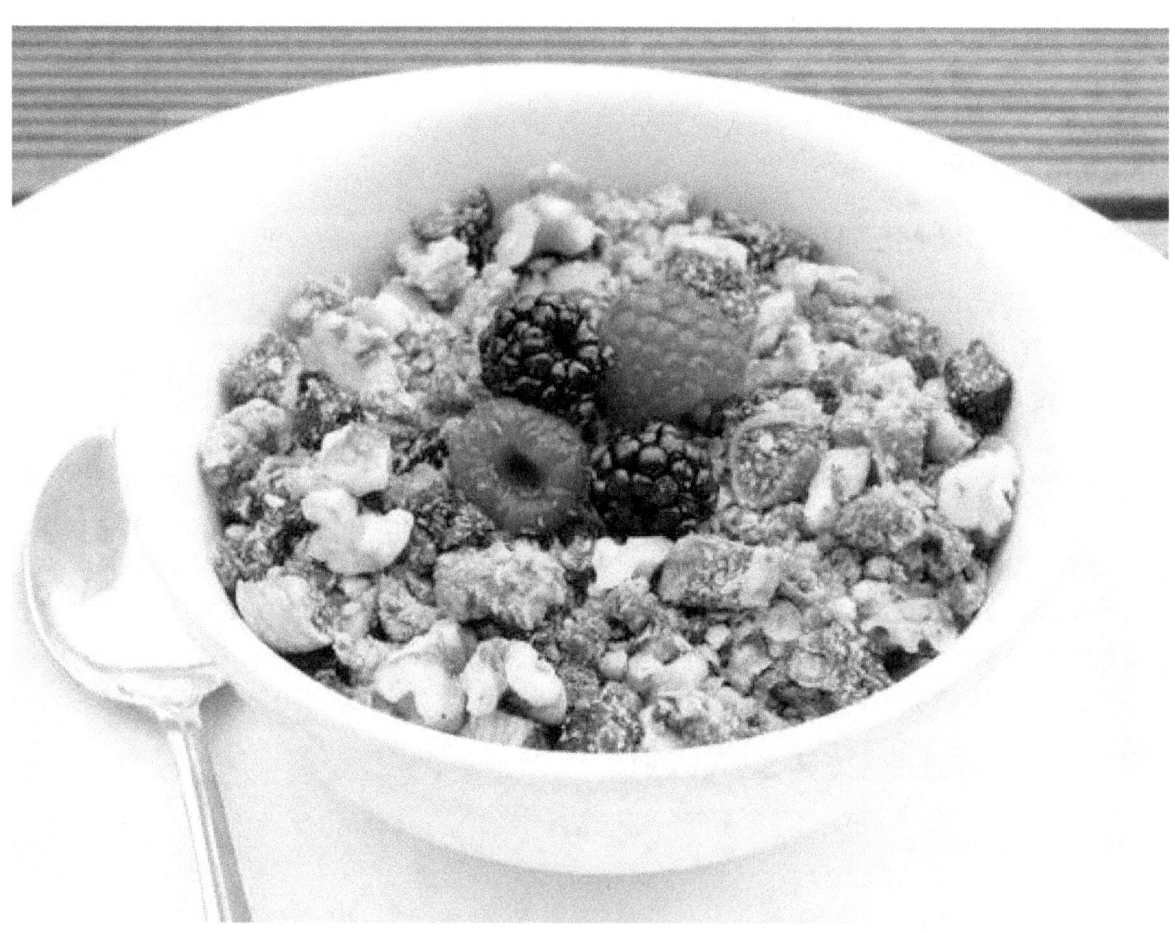

INGREDIENTS

¼ cup dried apricots

¼ cup dried cranberries

¼ cup shelled pumpkin seeds

¼ roasted almonds

¼ tsp kosher salt

½ cup flaxseed meal

1 ½ cup oats

1 cup barley flakes

1 cup rye flakes

PREPARATION METHOD

1. Mix all ingredients in a bowl and serve fresh

NUTRIENT VALUE PER SERVING

Calories: 260 Kcal

Fat: 9g

Carbohydrates: 39g

Protein: 10.5g

ARUGULA AND ROASTED CHICKPEA SALAD WITH FETA

SERVING SIZE

4 persons

COOKING TIME

20 minutes

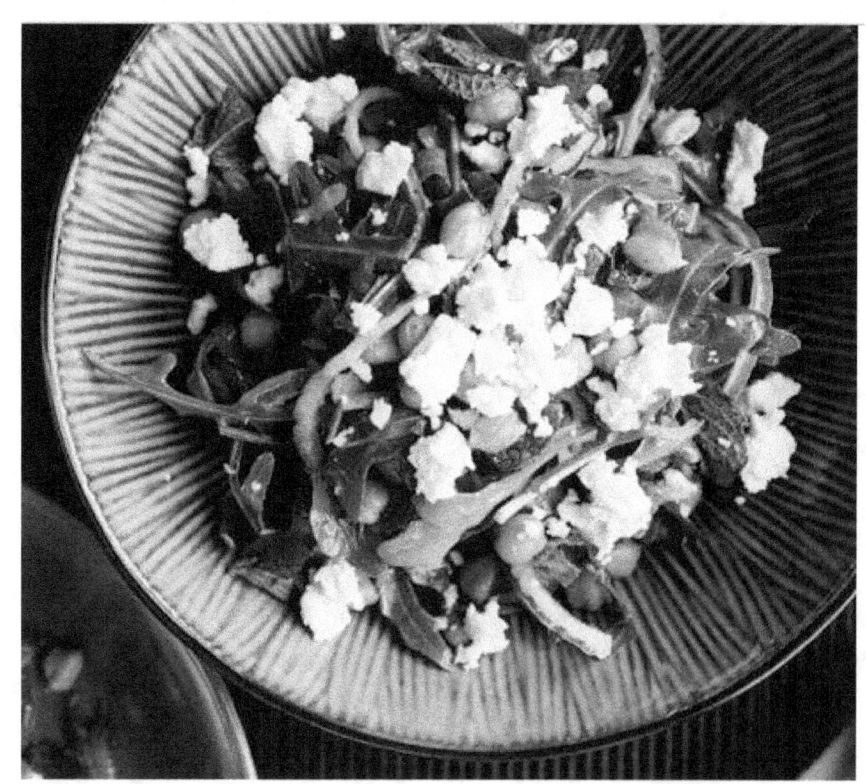

INGREDIENTS

112 ounce chickpeas

¼ cup mint leaves

¼ cup sliced red onions

1 tbsp lemon juice

1 tsp vinegar

2 tsp mint

3 ounce feta cheese

5 ounce arugula

5 tbsp olive oil

Kosher salt and black pepper

PREPARATION METHOD

1. Bake half chickpeas drizzled with oil and seasoned with salt and pepper in preheated oven at 400 degrees, until golden brown. Set aside to cool
2. In a bowl whisk 3 tbsp oil, 1 tbsp lemon juice, dried mint and vinegar. Season with salt and pepper
3. Combine arugula, fresh mint, remaining chickpeas and onion in bowl and toss gently.
4. Divide salad in plates, topped with roasted chickpeas and feta

NUTRIENT VALUE PER SERVING

Calories: 280 Kcal

Fat: 5g

Carbohydrates: 14g

Protein: 9g

KALE SALAD AND BUTTERNUT SQUASH AND ALMONDS

SERVING SIZE

4 persons

COOKING TIME

40 minutes

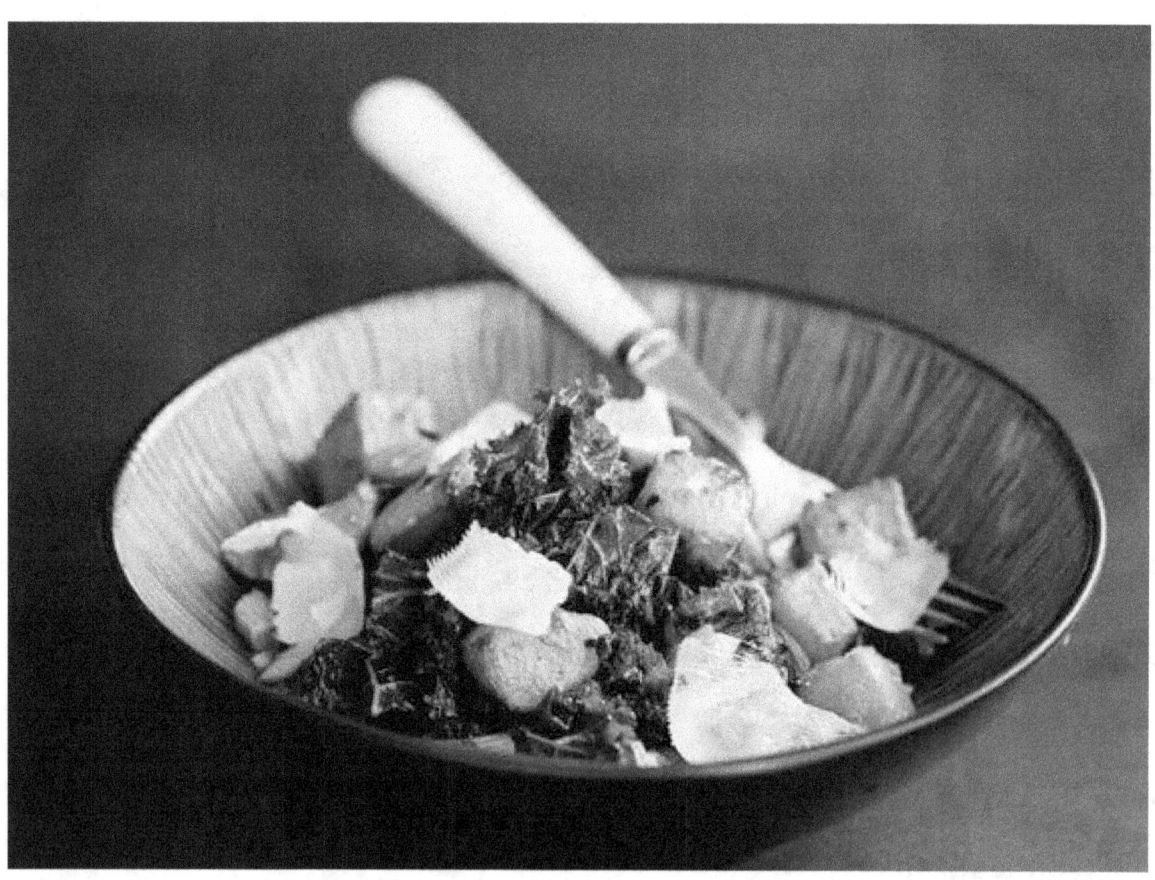

INGREDIENTS

8 tbsp olive oil

3 tbsp vinegar

½ minced shallot

1 tsp mustard

Kosher salt and black pepper

1 ½ cup cubed butternut squash

I bunch kale

¾ cup toasted almonds

Parmesan

PREPARATION METHOD

1. Preheat oven to 450 degrees
2. In a bowl whisk 5 tbsp oil, vinegar, shallot and mustard, season with salt and pepper and set aside
3. In another bowl combine squash and 2 tbsp oil and transfer to baking sheet to roast until lightly brown. Set aside to cool
4. Heat 1 tbsp oil in skillet and add kale and cook for 2 minutes. Remove from heat and add 4 tbsp dressing and toss. Transfer kale to baking sheet and let it cool.
5. Toss reserved squash and almonds with kale and season with pepper. Drizzle with parmesan and remaining dressing. Divide in plates and serve.

NUTRIENT VALUE PER SERVING

Calories: 500 Kcal

Fat: 6g

Carbohydrates: 25g

Protein: 11g

CIDER-GLAZED CHICKEN BREASTS WITH APPLE-FENNEL SALAD

SERVING SIZE

Serves 4

COOKING TIME

45 minutes

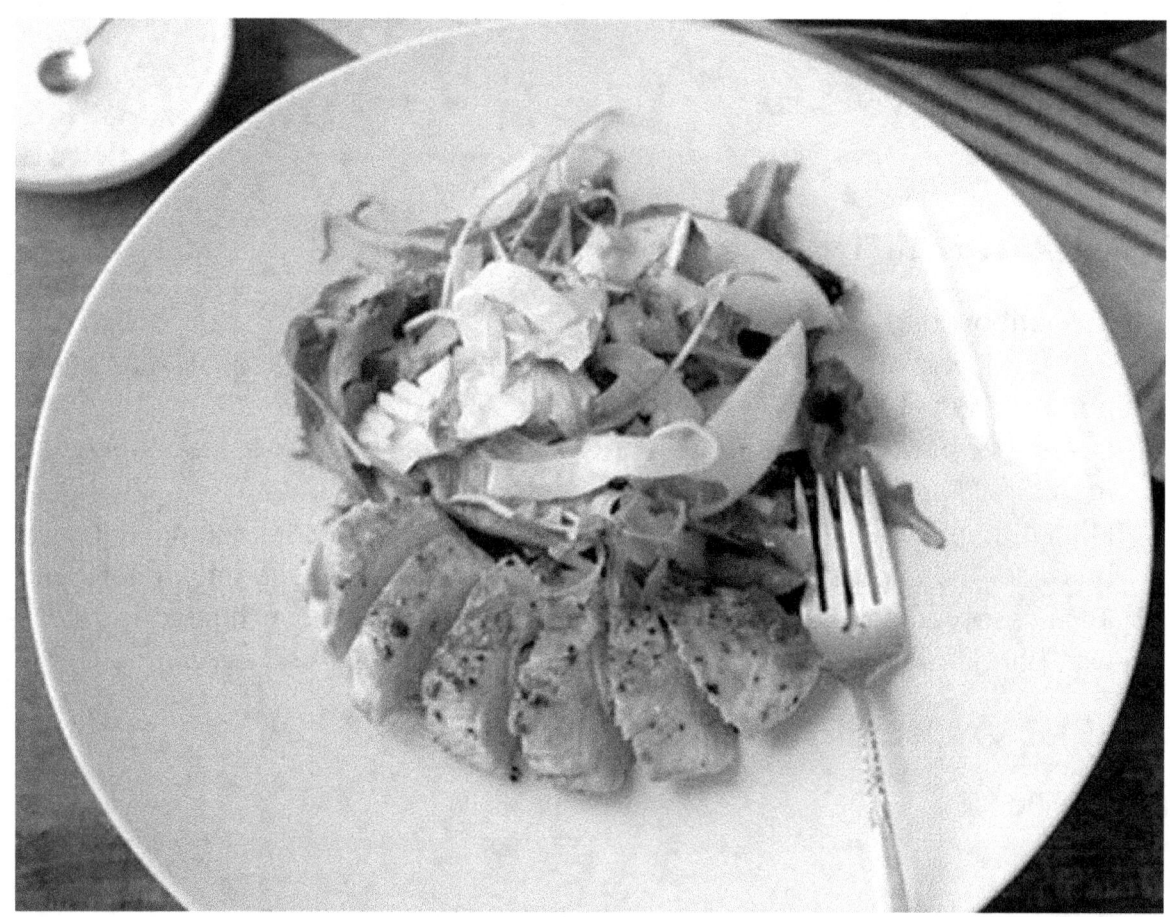

INGREDIENTS

4 boneless chicken breasts

Kosher salt and black pepper

½ apple

½ finely chopped shallot

3 tbsp apple cider vinegar

2/4 tsp mustard powder

5 tbsp oil

½ cup apple cider

1 tbsp unsalted butter

4 cups baby lettuce

½ thinly sliced fennel bulb

PREPARATION METHOD

1. Preheat oven to 400 degree and season chicken breasts with salt and pepper
2. Chop one apple slice and add with shallot, 2 tbsp cider vinegar and mustard in bowl. Whisk in 3 tbsp oil after 10 minutes.
3. Heat 2 tbsp oil in skillet and cook chicken until golden brown. Transfer skillet to oven and cook for 15 minutes. Put chicken on plate
4. Add cider to skillet over medium high heat and boil until it is reduced to half. Add 1 tbsp vinegar. Add butter after removing from heat and season with cider sauce and salt
5. Slice the remaining apple and add it to a bowl with lettuce and fennel. Season with salt and pepper to taste. Divide it with the chicken in plates and serve with sauce.

NUTRIENT VALUE PER SERVING

Calories: 419.7

Fat: 52.5g

Carbohydrates: 6.8g

Protein: 41.2

CRISPY KALE SALAD WITH LIME DRESSING

SERVING SIZE

Serves 6

COOKING TIME

40 minutes

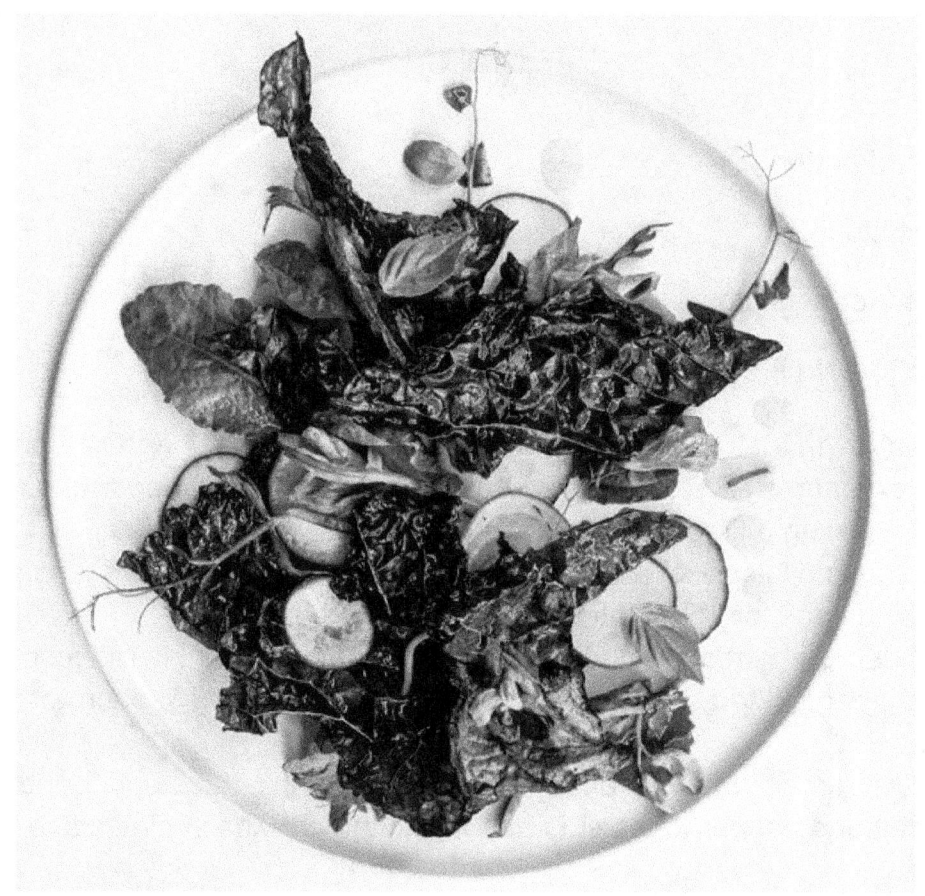

INGREDIENTS

1 ½ tbsp sugar

¼ cup lime

3 tbsp fish sauce

1 tsp minced garlic

½ red chili

24 tuscan kale leaves

1 tbsp oil

Salt and pepper

3 cups of mixed basil, mint and cilantro

3 cups of mixed carrots, beets and radishes

2 cups pea tendrils

1 cup sliced cucumber

PREPARATION METHOD

1. Dissolve sugar in 2 tbsp water and cool it. Mix in lime juice, fish sauce, garlic and red chili for dressing and set aside.
2. Preheat oven to 250 degrees. Bake kale leaves seasoned with oil and salt and pepper for 30 minutes until crisp.
3. Mix the remaining ingredients with the dressing. Divide into plates and serve topped with crispy kale leaves.

NUTRIENT VALUE PER SERVING

Calories: 90 Kcal

Fat: 3g

Carbohydrates: 14g

Protein: 3g

EGGPLANT AND BEEF STIR-FRY

SERVING SIZE

Serves 4

COOKING TIME

30 minutes

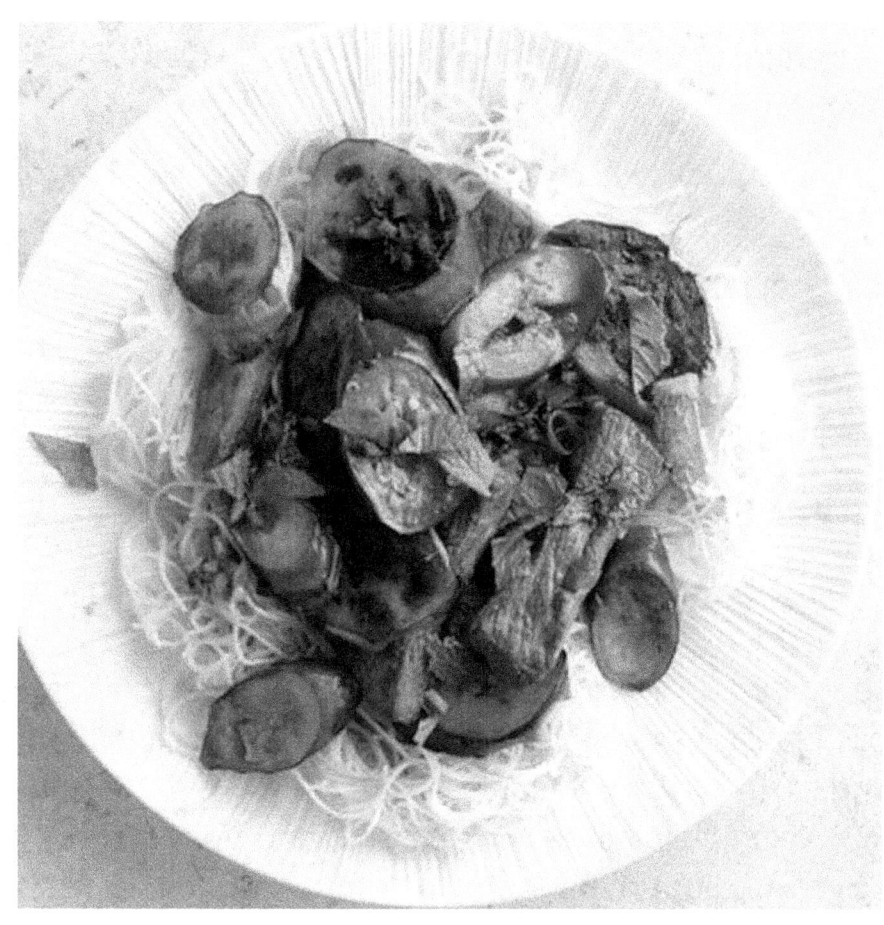

INGREDIENTS

4 tbsp chopped mint

3 tbsp soy sauce

2 thai chilies

1 thinly sliced ginger

1 tbsp fish sauce

2 tbsp lime juice

½ tsp sugar

2 tsp minced garlic

¼ tsp sugar

5 tbsp oil

1 pound baby eggplant

½ pound beef

Steamed brown rice

PREPARATION METHOD

1. In a medium bowl, whisk 2 tbsp mint, soy sauce, 1 chili, half ginger, lime juice, 1 tsp garlic, sugar and 2 tbsp water.
2. Cook eggplant until golden brown on skillet over medium heat. Add 2 tbsp oil. Transfer the eggplant to a bowl and mix it with half of the dressing.
3. Add remaining chili, ginger, 1 tsp garlic and beef with 1 tbsp oil in skillet over medium-high heat. Cook for 3 minutes until beef is nicely seared. Add eggplant mixture and toss the mixture well.
4. Divide rice in bowls and serve with the dressing and stir-fry. Garnish with mint.

NUTRIENT VALUE PER SERVING

Calories: 502.6 Kcal

Fat: 23.7g

Carbohydrates: 54.1g

Protein: 19.4g